Ketogenic Diet For Beginners

The Step By Step Guide With 110 High-Fat Recipes And 7 Day Meal Plan For Weight Loss & Healthy Living

REID WELLS

ISBN-13:978-1976373114
ISBN-10:1976373115

DEDICATION

To Sadie, you're the best!

TABLE OF CONTENTS

INTRODUCTION

Overview Of The Keto Diet

The ketogenic diet was first designed as a treatment for childhood epilepsy. Researchers at Johns Hopkins Medical Center diet saw that fasting helped improve the amount of seizures epileptic patients had. Since it was not possible to go on extended periods of fasting, a diet was consequently developed to make the body think that it was in a state of fasting. Research established that a diet that is low in carbohydrate, high in fat, and providing the minimal protein necessary for growth could maintain starvation ketosis for extended periods of time.

And this is how the ketogenic diet came to be. The keto diet, as it is also known, is an extremely low-carbohydrate, high-fat diet with moderate amounts of protein that turns the body into a fat-burning machine. It is based on the principle that by restricting carbohydrates to a certain level, your body is pushed into a metabolic state known as ketosis, where it break the fat molecules down into ketones to use as alternative energy source.

'But I am not epileptic', someone may say, 'so why do I need this diet?' The keto diet offers tremendous health benefits as you would soon see below. It aids weight loss. It helps to maintain blood sugar levels, thereby providing diabetic individuals quick recovering from their conditions. It improves cholesterol levels. It helps to treat and prevent cancer. It also increases energy levels due to its fat-based meals. Keto means you will never again feel deprived as you can kiss the hunger and cravings goodbye!

Individuals who are considering low carbohydrate approaches to dieting will be interested in this diet as it bears similarity to other strict low-carbohydrate diets such as the Atkins diet. However, the main difference is that protein is restricted in the keto diet. There are also others: ketogenic diet will not lead to muscle loss. You burn fat without sacrificing muscle, which makes you look lean and fit. This is great news for bodybuilders, don't you think? Fitness and bikini models can also use this diet on pre-competition.

KETO DIET BENEFITS

Being on a low-carb, high-fat diet comes with numerous benefits as mentioned earlier. Let's consider a few:

<u>Weight Loss</u>

The ketogenic diet basically uses body fat as an energy source. This is because of the significant drop in the insulin (the hormone responsible for storing fat) levels. Consequently, your body begins to burn its own stored fat for energy, leading to weight loss. Unlike starvation, that often leads to large loss of body protein, mainly from muscle tissue, the keto diet provides quick and easy weight loss, while allowing dieters to eat as much fat as they desire with minimal protein.

This makes weight loss a significant benefit of the ketogenic diet on account of the lower insulin levels and the body's act of burning stored fat. The aim of this diet for weight loss is 'eat fat to lose fat'. Consequently, you will record weight loss every single week of being on the diet, particularly in the first month. You will not be bothered about regaining your lost weight as long as you stick to the keto diet formula of eating high fat, low carb and moderate proteins. Additionally, some blood pressure issues are linked with excess weight, which is a good thing since keto leads to weight loss

Control Blood Sugar

Since the keto diet is selective on the kind of foods to eat, it naturally results in lower blood sugar levels. Studies have shown that this diet compared to low-calorie diets is better at managing and preventing diabetes. Individuals, who are type 2 diabetes but who aren't on insulin, can benefit from the ketogenic diet.

Mental Focus

If you are thinking of increasing your mental performance, consider the ketogenic diet. Ketones, product of this diet, are very good for the brain. Also, lowering carb intake makes it possible to avoid increase in blood sugar which helps you to focus and concentrate significantly.

Normalized Hunger & Increased Energy

Other diets make people feel miserable due to hunger and they eventually give up. But with the low carb, high fat diet, you experience an automatic reduction in appetite; you will eat fewer calories effortlessly and surprisingly feel satisfied. Additionally, you can say good-bye to ups and downs. With the keto diet, you will notice stability in your energy levels. You will always have a full tank of energy to run your day. Your physical performance will be enhanced.

Cholesterol Benefits

Although the ketogenic diet is high in fat, it won't raise your cholesterol or increase your risk for heart disease. This is because the fats are heart-healthy fats or 'good fats' and not trans fats that may lead to inflammation which causes heart disease. The keto diet leads to a significant increase in blood levels of HDL.

Improved Skin Condition

It's common to experience improvements in your skin when you switch to a ketogenic diet. Studies have shown an improvement in acne, skin inflammations and lesions.

For most people, the keto diet is safe. However, people on diabetes medication, especially those on insulin need to consult their doctor because their insulin dosages will need to be adjusted. Also, the keto diet is not considered safe pregnant and nursing mothers as well those with those with high blood pressure.

How The Keto Diet Works

The main source of energy for the body is glucose and this glucose is derived from the breakdown of carbohydrates that we consume in our diet. As long as it's available, the body will use it first, since it's the quickest to metabolize. However, when your body doesn't have enough carbs for the energy that's needed, it will start to burn fat. The aim of the ketogenic diet is to cause the body to burn fat as its primary source. This is why we limit carbohydrate intake as much as possible to prevent the body from using it as energy's primary source but to burn stored fat instead.

Biologically, the human body has three storehouse of energy for use in times of caloric deficiency: carbohydrate, protein and fat. Carbohydrate is stored as glycogen in the muscle and liver; protein also, can be converted to glucose in the liver and used for energy; and fat is stored mainly as body fat. However, there is an alternative fuel for the body, called ketones, which is used only when blood sugar (glucose) is in short supply.

ALL forms of carbohydrates; be it grains, sugar, starchy foods, fruits and vegetables, are broken down into glucose and stored as glycogen in the body. Excess glycogen that isn't presently needed by the body for energy is stored in the liver and the muscles. If the liver and muscles are full, the excess glycogen is then converted into triglycerides (fat molecules) and stored in your blood. But, this is not good at all, as it can lead to heart disease. This is why when people on the keto diet restrict carb consumption; they reduce blood triglycerides significantly and consequently lower their risk of heart disease.

Now back to the main subject: Glucose can only be stored in our muscles and liver for 24 hours. After a while, the liver starts to produce ketones as the main fuel source for the body. Ketones or ketone bodies are generated from the breakdown of fatty acids in the liver when glucose becomes unavailable. Ketones are in fact, produced in minute amounts whenever we go without food for several hours; for instance, after a full night's sleep. Nevertheless, the liver produces more ketones during fasting or when carbohydrate intake drops below 40 grams per day.

A keto diet is designed specifically to result in ketosis where your entire metabolism will switch over to using ketones as fuel instead of glucose. Remember, the golden formula of this diet is: Low carb, high fat and moderate protein.

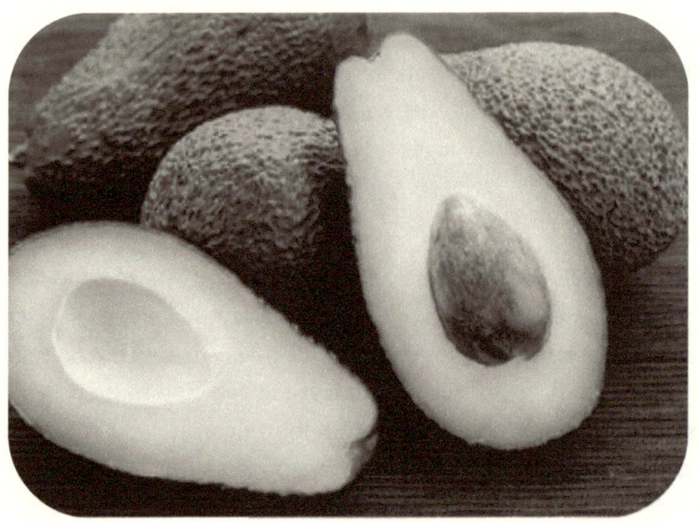

Adapting To Ketosis

During the ketosis phase, our body starts using Ketones as its energy source. It takes about 2 weeks of eating low carbohydrates foods for the body to adapt to this new course of metabolism. The carbohydrate must be quite low in quantity (20-30 gm of net carb per day) for this to happen. But, if you want to enter into ketosis within 1 week, you can cut your carbs to fewer than 15g per day.

Regardless of your body structure, you can be sure of attaining ketosis when you eat 20 grams of net carbs or less. As a matter of fact, our brain only requires 20-30grams of daily glucose to function well. Once you are keto-adapted, ketones becomes the main source of energy for the brain — up to 75%. Glucose becomes the secondary source, providing the remaining 25% energy needed by the brain. Therefore, when you eat 20-30g carbs, it will be used by your brain, especially when there is no stored glycogen in place. But if you eat more than 30 grams carbs, your muscles and your liver will begin to fill up with glycogen which impedes the benefits of ketosis.

Now during these two weeks of entering ketosis, you will experience some symptoms known as the 'keto flu' which includes headaches, brain fogginess, fatigue and sluggishness. These issues will however be corrected with proper electrolyte intake. The ketogenic diet is a natural diuretic, making you pee more than normal, so make sure you drink lots of water and take lots of salt. Drink at least 4 liters of water per day. It makes it easier if you add a little salt in it. This should help with the headaches. You're peeing out electrolytes, hence the thumping headaches. The water and salt intake will enable your body to re-hydrate and replenish your electrolytes.

A significant loss of water is often experienced in the first phases of ketosis. Remember that carbs are converted to glycogen in the body and stored inside water which is located within the liver and muscles. Your body flushes this water out as you use up stored glycogen. The result of this is a significant weight loss during the initial few weeks of ketosis. Additionally, do not worry about caloric restriction within these two weeks. For when you are in ketosis, your cravings for sugar and processed food reduces. You feel strong and have lots of energy. Consequently, weight loss will occur.

CALORIES & MACRONUTRIENTS

A calorie is a unit of energy. A meal containing 100 calories, for instance, indicates the amount of energy your body will get from eating that meal. The amount of calorie a person consumes determines the weight gain or loss. If you consume less calorie than you burn, you are likely to lose weight. Then again, if you do not eat the right calories, you may end up losing muscles as well. One way to guarantee that you are eating correctly is to count macros. It is much better to count macros than calories. An avocado that contains 100 calories (fat), for instance, will steer you towards your ketogenic goal than a doughnut containing 100 calories (carb)

Macros, short for macronutrients are what constitute the food we eat each day– primarily carbohydrates, fat and protein. They are needed by the body in large amounts and are measured in grams (g) on nutritional labels. To count macros, simply add up the number of grams of carbs, fats and protein that you ate that day.

Carbs: 1 gram of carbohydrates provides 4 calories

Fat: 1 gram of fat provides 9 calories

Protein: 1 gram of carbohydrates provides 4 calories

In the keto diet, the percentage of the calories that you eat should come from about 70-75 % fat, 20-25% protein and 5% carb. However this percentage varies from person to person as it depends on current lean body weight, daily activity level and goals.

To determine the precise carb count that's appropriate for you, you'll have to work out your total daily calorie intake. Search online for ketogenic-based macro calculators where you can easily enter in your numbers and get a quick estimation of your body's caloric needs and to find out your best percentages for each macronutrient.

Have it in mind that if you go beyond your macros with protein, you will be out of ketosis. This is the reason you must monitor your protein consumption while on the keto diet. The protein macros should not be above 0.8 gm per pound of body weight. This will prevent the central nervous system from making a quick metabolism switch to glucose when there is a variation in the ratio of carbs, fats and proteins.

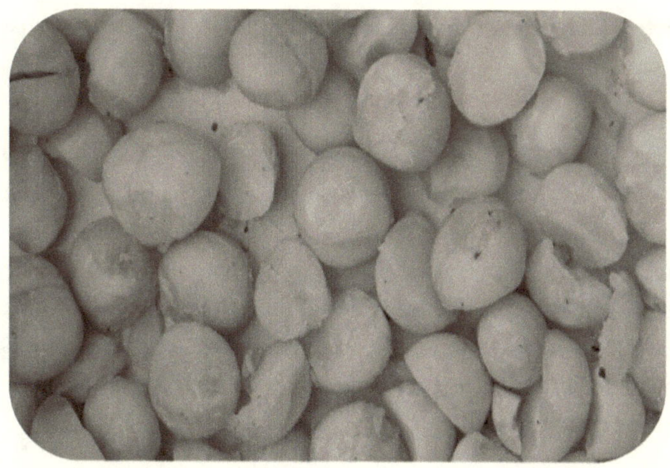

Nuts

KETO-ADAPTING TIPS

Here are a few tips to remember on becoming keto-adapted:

1. **Lower your carb intake** to 15- 20 digestible grams per day. You do not have to restrict fiber. It might even be beneficial.

2. **Eat moderate amount of protein**. If you can, restrict your intake to1 gram protein per day, per 1kg of body weight. So if you weigh 70 kilos (154 lbs.), consume about 70 grams of protein. If overweight, lower your protein consumption even more. Do not make the common mistake of consuming too much protein and thus hinder your optimal ketosis goal. This is because if your carb intake is low but your protein intake is high, the body will break down the amino acids that are present in protein for energy. This is known as gluconeogenesis.

3. To prevent this from happening, **keep your fat intake high** so your body can utilizes it and ketones for energy instead. Eat enough fat to feel satisfied. Ketogenic diet isn't starvation. A ketogenic diet is sustainable, starvation is not.

4. **Drink MCT Oil**. MCT (medium chain triglycerides) oil is unlike other fats. For one thing, it is one of the quickest energy sources that is absorbed quickly into the body, goes directly to the liver and immediately converts to energy in the form of ketones. MCT oil makes it possible to take in extra protein and carbs while keeping up with the ketogenic state. Beginners on keto diet will find it very rewarding. To use this oil, simply add to a cup of coffee or tea, mix and enjoy.

5. **Stay Hydrated**. As mentioned earlier, you will experience lower insulin level while on this diet, causing your kidneys to excrete a larger quantity of water and sodium. Therefore, drink water a lot to beat dehydration. How

frequent? Once you wake up in the morning and about 32 to 48 oz of water before noon. As a rule, drink at least 1/2 of what you weigh in ounces every day. So if you weigh 200 lbs., you should drink no less than 100 ounces of water in a day. However, if you exercise or sweat a lot, drink more!

6. **Consume Enough Quality Salts**. While on the ketogenic diet, you will be excreting more sodium. Consequently, you will need to consume more salt. Go for quality salt like the Pink Himalayan sea salt. A teaspoon is equal 2 grams of sodium. You need about 3 to 5 grams of sodium every day. You can get this from natural foods that are rich in sodium such as:

- sprouted and salted pumpkin seeds

- salted macadamia nuts

- broth

- low carb foods that contain sodium such as celery and cucumbers

- bacon and pickled vegetables

7. **Up Your Activity Level**. Perform regular exercises as this has been proven to moderately increase ketones levels while depleting glucogen reserves. There are high intensity exercises like squats, deadlifts, push-ups and pull-offs that can help to speed up the glucose transport molecule (GLUT-4 receptor) that are located within in the liver as well as muscle tissue. But you could also engage in low intensity exercises such as swimming, walking and slow jogging.

8. **Get Quality Sleep**. It is important to get quality sleep. If you don't, you may raise your stress hormones and this will increase your blood sugar. Try to get about 7 hours of sleep each night. The more stress you are, the more sleep you need.

9. **Take Supplement exogenous ketones**. However, this is usually not necessary.

Exogenous ketones are originally made for keto-adapted athletes or bodybuilders to make them perform better. It was also designed for people with neurological disorders such as epilepsy. Do not give in to the pressure to buy exogenous ketones. You can still get the energy level that you desire with a proper hydration.

Taking exogenous ketones artificially raises your ketone bodies, putting you in a ketosis state even if you've just had a high-carb meal. Most of these exogenous ketones will be excreted through the urine and none of them may be used to burn fat. Nevertheless, if you really want to try exogenous ketones, ensure you research the product you wish to buy thoroughly and be sure it is third-party-tested and uses first-rate materials.

Measuring Your Ketosis

To reach ketosis, you will have to be diligent about knowing the carb count that your body needs. The good news about ketosis is that it is measurable. You can always measure your metabolic state to ascertain where you stand. Even when you have determined your perfect amount of carb by determining your total daily calorie intake, you still need to know whether your body is creating ketones by testing your ketones levels. There are a few ways to do this

1. **Check How You Feel**

Keto dieters, due to low sodium levels will experience flu-like symptoms that include headaches, fatigue, irritability, cough, sniffles and nausea. These symptoms, due to electrolyte imbalances, come with starting keto.

2. **Use Urine Ketone Strips**

This is simple and affordable, and a common option for many beginners. They are available in regular pharmacies and online stores. Simple dip the stick in a sample of your urine, wait 15 minutes and then view for color change. If it is dark purple in color, then you are in ketosis.

The disadvantage of this is that the results may vary due to the quantity of liquid that you drink. The more keto-adapted you are, the more your body reabsorbs ketones from the urine. The urine strips will no longer be effective as it will keep reading negative, even when you have been in ketosis for some time. As mentioned earlier, it is only good for beginners.

3. Breath-ketone analyzers

These are more reliable than the urine strips, though a bit costlier. They are reusable as well. While they do not give you an accurate ketone level, they provide a color code for the general level. However, there are not portable, as they require computer hookup to read. They are also not totally accurate and may sometimes show values that are completely misleading.

4. **Blood-Ketone Meters**

Blood-ketone meters are the best. They are reliable and show accurate readings. By using them, you are guaranteed of current ketone levels in your blood. However, they are quite costly.

The Keto Diet And What You Eat

Starting the ketogenic diet requires planning ahead. If you want to get into a ketogenic state quickly, you must be mindful of what you eat. The more you limit your carb intake to say, less than 15 grams a day, the quicker you will attain this state. The key features of a ketogenic diet are low amount of dietary carbohydrates and a high amount of dietary fat. The ratio of the diet is 75% dietary fat, 20% proteins and only 5% carbohydrates or around 70% fats, 25% protein, and 5% carbohydrate. However, this ratio can be adjusted for different people.

Your nutrient intake should be between 20 to 30g of net carbs per day. Net carbs are your total dietary carbohydrates, minus dietary fiber and sugar alcohols. Fiber and sugar alcohol do not raise blood sugar because they cannot be broken into glucose. Consequently, most people do not count them towards their total carb count. For example, if 1 cup of broccoli contains 6g of carb and 2 g fiber. The net carb of 1 cup broccoli will be 4g (having subtracted the dietary fiber from the total carb). For weight loss, it is advisable to monitor both your total carbs and net carbs. In most cases, a maximum of 20g carbohydrate for one day is all that's required for weight loss. The ketogenic diet work due to its restrictive nature and it will work for you as long as you weigh the carbohydrate and fat content of each food you eat.

So what to eat? A limited consumption of carbohydrate, of course! But to do this, eat mostly vegetables, dairy and nuts. Do not eat refined carbohydrates such as starch (legumes, beans and potatoes), wheat (pasta, bread cereals) and fruits. However, you can eat a moderate amount of berries, avocado and star fruit. You need foods that are high in dietary fat such as butter, ghee and coconut oil. Lean protein foods like chicken, eggs and fish are a must. Green vegetables like broccoli and spinach are essential in the ketogenic diet. It's really is simple: limit carbohydrate, consume protein as needed and fill up the rest of the calories with fat.

Fats: Fats are very important to the ketogenic diet. You can consume them in many different ways to add to your meals. Saturated fats like butter and gee are good. Monounsaturated fats like olive oil and macadamia nuts are good but avoid transfat or processed fats such as margarine. Salmon, tuna, trout and shellfish will give you a balanced diet of omega 3. Organic and grass-fed sources of fats and oils are preferable.

Protein: Go for pasture-raised and grass-fed protein to minimize bacteria. For poultry, the darker meat tends to be fattier, so go for these as well. Avoid the temptation of eating too much protein as it could cause a decrease in the production of ketone production and an increase in glucose production. Lamb is very fatty. If you don't eat beef and pork, you can go for lamb instead.

Vegetables And Fruit: Vegetables are important to a healthy keto diet. But be careful, some vegetables have sugar content. For the keto diet, you need vegetables with high nutrient content but low carb content. These vegetables are often dark and leafy such as spinach or kale. You can also try veggies that grow above ground but if you must eat vegetables that grow below ground such as onions, use for flavor and eat in moderation.

Dairy Products: Diary is a good way of adding extra fats too your diet. With dairy, you can create sauces or fatty side dishes. But consume diary moderately, as they contain protein as well. Go for raw and organic dairy products, if possible.

Highly processed dairy usually have higher fat content. It is also advisable to go for full fat products over fat-free or low-fat because they will have more quality carbs and less "filling" effects. The following dairy products are keto-compliant:

- Greek Yogurt
- Homemade Mayonnaise

- Heavy whipping cream
- Soft Cheese like Monterey jack, mozzarella, Colby, brie etc
- Hard Cheese like parmesan, aged cheddar, Swiss, feta, etc.
- Spread-ables such as cottage cheese, sour cream, cream cheese, crème fraiche, mascarpone, etc.

Water And Beverages

You need to lots of water on the keto diet. Drink about a gallon of water every day. Some examples of commonly consumed beverages on keto are below:

- Water: You need plenty of this; either still or sparkling water.

- Broth: one great way of replenishing your electrolytes.

- Coffee: beneficial for weight loss

- Tea: black or green tea is great.

- Alcohol: go for hard liquor and consume moderately.

General Products To Have

These basics in your home will guarantee healthy, keto-friendly meals at all times:

1. Fish and seafood

2. Low-carb vegetables (asparagus, broccoli, mushrooms, lettuce, cucumber, onions, cauliflower, peppers, garlic, tomatoes, zucchini, Brussels sprouts, etc.)

3. Cheese

4. Avocados

5. Meat and poultry

6. Eggs

7. Coconut oil

8. Plain Greek yoghurt and cottage cheese

9. Nuts and seeds (flaxseeds, chia seeds, macadamias, almonds, pecans, walnuts, etc.)

10. Olive oil

11. Berries

12. Butters and cream

13. Dark chocolate and cocoa

14. Unsweetened coffee and tea

15. Olives

16. Berries – (moderate consumption of raspberries, blackberries, strawberries)

17. low-carb sweeteners – (Stevia, erythritol, etc)

18. Fats and Oils: (butter, Peanut Butter, olive oil, almond oil sesame oil, flaxseed oil, etc)

Avoid:

- Grains: Wheat, cereal, oats, rye, corn, rice, barley, pasta, bread etc

- Tubers: potato, yams, etc.

- Sugar: honey, agave, maple syrup, etc.

- Processed Foods containing carrageenan

- Fruit – apples, bananas, oranges, etc.

- Artificial Sweeteners: Sucralose, Saccharin, Splenda, etc.

- Diet soda

- Fat-free and low-fat dairy products including regular milk, skim milk and sweetened yogurts

- Beer

- donut

- candy/ chocolate bar

- etc

A 7-DAY KETO DIET MEAL PLAN

DAY 1

<u>Breakfast</u>

<u>Chia Mocha Pudding</u>

<u>Lunch</u>

<u>Asian Broccoli Salad</u>

<u>Dinner</u>

<u>Lobster Bisque</u>

DAY2

<u>Breakfast</u>

<u>Keto Scrambled Eggs Recipe</u>

<u>Lunch</u>

<u>Meatloaf Cupcakes</u>

<u>Dinner</u>

Cauliflower Tabbouleh

Preparation time: 5 minutes

Cooking time: 0 minutes

Servings: 2

Ingredients:

3.5 oz of cauliflower florets

2 tbsp parsley, diced finely

3 mint leaves, diced finely

1 slice lemon diced

2 cherry tomatoes, diced

1 tbsp olive oil

Salt and pepper to taste

Directions:

1. In a food processor, process the cauliflower florets so that the texture is couscous- like. Prior to processing, ensure the processor and florets are dry to prevent it from being mashy.

2. Now combine the processed products and the herbs, lemon slice, tomatoes, olive oil, salt and pepper, mixing well.

Nutritional Information Per Serving (Serving size: 90 g)

Calories - 80, Carbohydrates – 5g, Fat - 7g, Proteins- 1g, Fiber - 2g

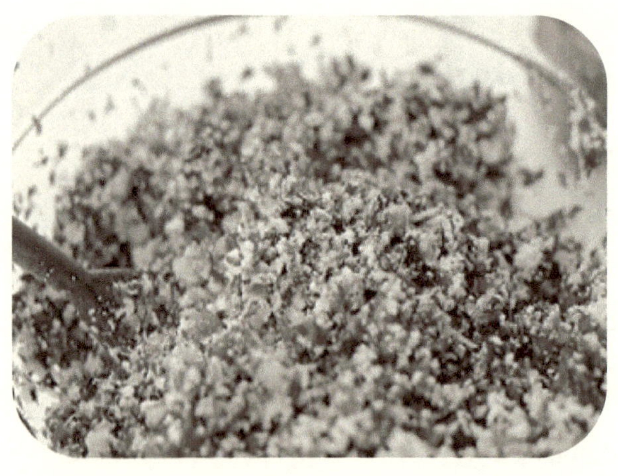

<u>Snack</u>

<u>Caprese Meatballs</u>

DAY 3

<u>Breakfast</u>

<u>Keto Breakfast Brownie Muffins</u>

<u>Lunch</u>

Mustard Sardines Salad

Preparation time: 5 minutes

Cooking time: 0 minutes

Servings: 1

Ingredients:

1 can (4 to5 oz) sardines in olive oil

¼ cucumber, peeled & diced a little

1 tbsp lemon juice

½ tbsp mustard

Salt & pepper to taste

Directions:

1. Drain the olive oil from the sardines, leaving just a little

2. Mash the sardines up.

3. Combine the sardines with the rest of the ingredients, mixing well.

Nutritional Information Per Serving

Calories -260, Carbohydrates – 0g, Fat - 20g, Proteins- 25g,

Dinner

Beef Chili

DAY 4

Breakfast

Green Keto Smoothie

Lunch

Chicken Dill Salad

Dinner

Turkey Meatballs In Curry Sauce

DAY5

Breakfast

Keto Pumpkin Spiced Granola

Lunch

Broccoli Bacon Salad With Onions And Coconut Cream

Preparation time: 5 minutes

Cooking time: 10 minutes

Servings: 6

Ingredients:

1 lb broccoli florets

4 small red onions or 2 large ones, sliced

20 slices of bacon, chopped into small pieces

1 cup coconut cream

Salt to taste

Directions:

1. Begin by cooking the bacon and then add the onions and cook.

2. Blanche the broccoli florets or use raw.

3. Add together the onions, bacon pieces, broccoli florets with the coconut cream and then season with salt.

Nutritional Information Per Serving (serving size: 1 bowl)

Calories - 280, Carbohydrates – 8g, Fat - 26g, Proteins- 7g, Fiber - 3g

Dinner

Turkey And Bacon Chowder

DAY 6

Breakfast

Egg Porridge

Lunch

Keto Cabbage Slaw

Dinner

Chinese Pulled Pork

DAY 7

<u>Breakfast Waffles</u>

<u>Lunch</u>

Zucchini Beef Sauté With Cilantro& Garlic

Preparation time: 5 minutes

Cooking time: 15 minutes

Servings: 2

Ingredients:

10 oz beef, sliced into strips of ½ inches

1 zucchini, cut into strips of 1-2 inch in length

¼ cup cilantro, chopped

3 cloves of garlic, minced or diced

2 tbsp tamari sauce, gluten-free

Avocado, coconut or olive oil for cooking

Directions:

1. In a pan, sauté the beef strips in 2 tablespoons oil for a 2-4 minutes on high heat.

2. Once browned, add the zucchini strips and sauté until zucchini is soft.

3. Add the garlic, tamari sauce and cilantro.

4. Sauté another few minutes and then serve immediately.

Nutritional Information Per Serving

Calories – 500, Carbohydrates – 5g, Fat - 40g, Proteins- 31g, Fiber -1g

<u>Dinner</u>

<u>Creamed Lemon Mustard Pork Loin</u>

BREAKFAST AND SMOOTHIES

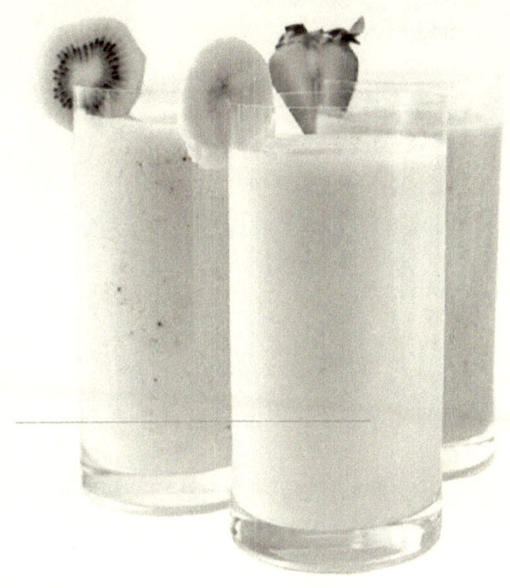

Egg Porridge

Start your day on a sweet and creamy note.

Preparation time: 5 minutes

Cooking time: 10 minutes

Servings: 1

Ingredients:

1/3 cup of organic heavy cream

2 eggs

2 packages of sweetener

2 tablespoons of butter

Ground Ceylon cinnamon

Directions:

1. In a small bowl, whisk the cream, eggs and sweetener.

2. In a medium sauce pan, melt the butter over medium high heat. Ensure that the color does not turn to brown.

3. Add the cream mixture to the pan and cook until the mixture becomes thick and starts to curdle.

4. Remove from heat, put in a serving dish, sprinkle lots of cinnamon on it and serve.

Nutritional Information Per Serving

Calories - 661, Carbohydrates - 2.9g, Fat - 64.5g, Proteins -17.3g

Chia Mocha Pudding

Breakfast does not get healthier than this.

Preparation time: 5 minutes

Cooking time: 30 minutes

Servings: 2

Ingredients:

1/3 cup of undiluted coconut cream

1/3 cup of dry chia seeds

2 tablespoons of cacao nibs

2 tablespoons of herbal coffee

1 tablespoon of swerve

1 tablespoon of vanilla extract

Directions:

1. Simmer 2 cups of water with the herbal coffee for 15 minutes to brew a strong coffee. Strain the coffee.

2. Add the vanilla extract, coconut cream and swerve to the coffee and blend together.

3. Add the cacao nibs and chia seeds. Stir thoroughly to combine.

4. Chill in serving containers for a minimum of 30 minutes before serving.

Nutritional Information Per Serving

Calories - 257, Carbohydrates - 2.25g, Fats - 20.25g, Proteins - 7g, Fiber - 11.5g

Breakfast Waffles

It's literally grain and sugar free.

Preparation time: 10 minutes

Cooking time: 20 minutes

Servings: 5

Ingredients:

4 tablespoons of granulated sweetener

4 tablespoons of coconut flour

3 tablespoons of full fat milk

5 eggs separated

2 teaspoons of vanilla

1 teaspoon of baking powder

1 stick plus 1 tablespoon of melted butter

Directions:

1. Beat the egg whites in a bowl until it is firm and forms stiff peaks. Set aside.

2. In another bowl, combine the coconut flour, baking powder, egg yolks and sweetener. Slowly add the butter and mix until smooth.

3. Add the vanilla and milk. Thoroughly combine.

4. Fold spoons of the egg whites gently into the flour mixture.

5. Put the mixture into a warm waffle maker and cook until it turns golden.

Nutritional Information Per Serving

Calories - 280, Carbohydrates - 4.5g, Fat - 26g, Proteins - 7g, Fiber - 2g

Spicy Baked Granola
Simple to make and seriously filling.

Preparation time: 15 minutes

Cooking time: 1 hour 30 minutes

Servings: 4

Ingredients:

1 cup of pecans, chopped

1/2 cup of almond meal

1/2 cup of slivered almonds

1/2 cup of walnuts, chopped

1/2 cup of sweetener

1/2 cup of unsweetened flaked coconut

1/4 cup of water

1/4 cup of pumpkin seeds

1/4 cup of ground chia seeds or flax meal

1/4 cup of sunflower seeds

1/4 cup of butter, melted

1 teaspoon of vanilla

1 teaspoon of honey

1 teaspoon of cinnamon

1/2 teaspoon of nutmeg

1/2 teaspoon of salt

Directions:

1. Preheat oven to 250F.

2. Set a parchment paper piece on a baking sheet and grease it.

3. Thoroughly mix all the ingredients together in a large bowl and spread it on the baking sheet.

4. Set a second piece of parchment paper on the mixture and use a rolling pin to roll the mixture into an even and firm sheet. Discard the top piece of parchment paper.

5. Bake for 60-90 minutes or until it turns golden.

6. Cool completely before breaking into pieces.

Nutritional Information Per Serving

Calories - 765.77, Carbohydrates - 9.73g, Fat - 71.97g, Proteins - 20.29g, Fiber - 12.24g

Chive Cheddar Soufflés

Amazingly light, creamy and fabulous.

Preparation time: 10 minutes

Cooking time: 25 minutes

Servings: 8

Ingredients:

2 cups of sharp cheddar cheese, shredded

1/2 cup of almond flour

1/4 cup of fresh chives, chopped

3/4 cup of heavy cream

6 large eggs, separated

1 teaspoon of ground mustard

1 teaspoon of salt

1/2 teaspoon of xanthan gum

1/2 teaspoon of black pepper

1/4 teaspoon of cayenne pepper

1/4 teaspoon of cream of tartar

A dash of salt

Directions:

1. Preheat oven to 350F.

2. Grease 8 ramekins and place on a large cookie sheet.

3. Whisk the mustard, almond flour, cayenne, salt, xanthan gum and pepper
in a large bowl.

4. Whisk in the cream slowly until well mixed.

5. Whisk in the chives, egg yolks and cheese until it is fully combined.

6. Beat the egg whites with salt and the cream of tartar in a large bowl until it turns glossy and forms stiff peaks. Fold this mixture into the flour mixture carefully until it is thoroughly mixed.

7. Evenly divide the mixture between the ramekins and place in the oven.

8. Bake for about 25 minutes.

Nutritional Information Per Serving

Calories - 288, Carbohydrates - 3.32g, Fat - 23.60g, Proteins - 14.02g, Fiber - 1.01g

No-Dairy Green Smoothie
Drink your salad on the go.

Preparation time: 5 minutes

Cooking time: 0 minutes

Servings: 6

Ingredients:

4 cups of filtered water

1 cup of cucumber, raw, peeled & sliced

1 cup romaine lettuce

1/2 cup of peeled kiwi fruit, diced

1/3 cup of fresh pineapple, chopped

2 tablespoons of fresh parsley

1 tablespoon of fresh ginger, peeled and chopped

1 tablespoon of granulated sugar substitute

1/2 Hass avocado, pit removed and flesh scooped from shell

Directions:

Blend all the ingredients together in a blender until smooth.

Nutritional Information Per Serving

Calories - 37, Carbohydrates - 3g, Fat - 2g, Proteins - 1g

Green Keto Smoothie

Great for a quick and healthy breakfast

Preparation time: 2 minutes

Cooking time: 0 minutes

Servings: 1

Ingredients:

3 cups of water

2 cups of frozen spinach

2 tablespoons of chia seeds

2 tablespoons of flax meal

1 tablespoon of MCT oil

1 Scoop of whey protein

5 cubes of ice

Directions:

Blend all the ingredients on high speed for about 30 seconds until the spinach is mostly liquid.

Nutritional Information Per Serving

Calories - 485, Carbohydrates - 3g, Fat - 27g, Proteins - 40g, Fiber - 20g

Mint And Chocolate Smoothie

Just put it all in a blender.

Preparation time: 5 minutes

Cooking time: 0 minutes

Servings: 1

Ingredients:

1 cup of unsweetened cashew or almond milk

¼ cup of coconut milk

2 tablespoons of powdered erythriol or swerve

1 tablespoon of cocoa powder

1 tablespoon of MCT oil

½ medium avocado

A few leaves of fresh mint

A few ice cubes

Coconut milk or whipped cream, optional

Directions:

1. Blend all the ingredients together in a blender until smooth.

2. Top with the coconut milk or whipped cream if using.

Nutritional Information Per Serving

Calories - 401, Carbohydrates - 6.5g, Fat - 40.3g, Proteins - 5g, Fiber - 7.8g

Coffee Smoothie

Adds a wonderful perk to your mornings

Preparation time: 1 minute

Cooking time: 0 minutes

Servings: 2

Ingredients:

16 ounces of ice

6 ounces of cold coffee

4 ounces of unsweetened almond milk

4 ounces of heavy cream

1 ounce of sugar free caramel syrup

1 ounce of sugar free chocolate syrup

2 tablespoons of unsweetened cocoa

Directions:

Blend all the ingredients together in a blender until smooth.

Nutritional Information Per Serving

Calories - 216, Carbohydrates - 6g, Fat - 22g, Proteins - 3g, Fiber - 2g

Blackcurrant Strawberry Smoothie

Perfect for hot summer afternoons

Preparation time: 5 minutes

Cooking time: 0 minutes

Servings: 1

Ingredients:

½ cup of fresh or frozen blackcurrants

1/2 cup of water

¼ cup of heavy whipping cream or coconut milk

¼ cup of strawberries

2 tablespoons of whole or powdered chia seeds

½ vanilla bean

5-7 drops of liquid Stevia extract, optional

Directions:

1. Blend all the ingredients together in a blender until smooth.

2. Let it stand for 2-5 minutes

Nutritional Information Per Serving

Calories - 228, Carbohydrates - 8.7g, Fat - 17.3g, Proteins - 5.1g, Fiber - 9.4g

Keto Pumpkin Spiced Granola

Granola pairs well with cream, coconut milk, full-fat yogurt or almond milk and topped with berries.

Preparation Time: 30 minutes

Hands-on: 10 minutes

Servings: 8

Ingredients:

<u>Dry:</u>

1 cup whole almonds

½ cup pecan nuts

½ cup macadamia nuts

1 cup shredded dried coconut

½ cup pumpkin seeds

1 cup dried coconut, flaked

¼ cup chia seeds, whole or ground

½ cup vanilla or plain whey protein

¼ cup Erythritol

¼ tsp salt

1 tbsp+ 1 tsp homemade pumpkin pie spice mix

<u>Wet:</u>

1 large egg white

½ cup pumpkin puree

¼ cup extra virgin coconut oil, melted

10-15 drops liquid Stevia extract

Directions:

1. Preheat oven to 300 F. Chop the pecans, almonds and macadamia nuts and transfer to a mixing bowl. Add the flaked coconut, pumpkin seeds, chia seeds, protein powder and Erythritol.

2. Next, add the pumpkin spice mix and salt. Then the egg white, melted coconut oil and stevia. Mix well to combine.

3. Add the pumpkin puree, mix well then place the granola mixture on a baking tray, spreading over the surface evenly.

4. Bake in the oven for 30-40 minutes until crispy. remove from oven and set on a cooling rack.

5. Once chilled, remove to an airtight container at room temperature. Store for up to a month. Enjoy!

Nutritional Information Per Serving:

Calories: 434, Net Carbs: 5.6g, Total Carbs: 14.6g, Fats: 37.2g, Protein: 16g, Fiber: 9g

Bacon/ Avocado Breakfast

Preparation Time: 2 minutes

Cook Time: 10 minutes

Servings: 2

Ingredients:

4 strips bacon, uncured &pastured

1 large avocado, peeled & sliced

2 large organic eggs

¼ teaspoon Sea Salt

Directions

1. Add avocado and bacon to a pan on a medium flame and flip after 2-3 minutes.

2: Remove the avocado and bacon, set aside, keep warm but leave the drippings in the pan. Break eggs in the pan and fry 2-3 minutes

3. Flip the egg and fry to attain desired yolk consistency. Enjoy!

Nutritional Information Per Serving:

Calories: 313, Net Carbs: 2.5g, Fats: 26g, Protein: 13g, Fiber: 6g

Breakfast Brownie Muffins

Preparation Time: 15 minutes

Cook Time: 15 minutes

Servings: 6 Muffins

Ingredients:

1 cup Golden Flaxseed Meal

1 tbsp. Cinnamon

1/4 cup Cocoa Powder

1/2 tbsp. Baking Powder

1 large Egg

1/2 tsp. Salt

2 tbsp. Coconut Oil

1/4 cup Caramel Syrup, sugar-free

1/2 cup Pumpkin Puree

1 tsp. Apple Cider Vinegar

1 tsp. Vanilla Extract

1/4 cup Slivered Almonds

Directions

1. Preheat oven to 350°F. Combine all ingredients in a deep bowl and mix well to combine.

2. Line muffin tin with 6 paper liners and ladle ¼ cup of batter into each of the muffin liner.

3. Sprinkle slivered almonds over each muffin and gently press to make them adhere.

4. Bake about 15 minutes in the oven until muffins rise and set on top.

Nutritional Information Per Serving:

Calories: 183, Net Carbs: 3.3g, Fats: 13.4g, Protein: 7g,

\#

Extra- Rich High Fiber Cereal Breakfast

Try this crunchy-chocolaty Keto cereal With Cacao Nibs Keto and Low Carb juice, Cane Juice, Fruit-Juice Concentrate &Corn Sweetener. It is satisfying and full of beneficial fiber.

Preparation Time: 10 minutes

Cook Time: 1hour

Servings: 4

Ingredients:

1 cup water

4 tbsp hemp hearts

½ cup chia seeds

1 tbsp fine Psyllium powder

1 tbsp organic vanilla extract

2 tbsp coconut oil, melted

2 tbsp Raw Cacao Nibs

1 tbsp Swerve

Directions

1. Pre-heat oven to 285 degrees. Add the chia seeds and the water to a large mixing bowl and stir thoroughly to combine. Let it sit for about 5 minutes.

2. Add the remaining ingredients, except the cacao nibs, to the bowl. Mix all ingredients with a wooden spoon or an electric mixer, until evenly mixed.

3. (However, if you want your cacao nibs in bigger chunks do not add to the mix above, but add them now and stir into the dough)

4. Roll out two large pieces of parchment paper. Form the dough into a cylinder and place on the parchment paper with the shiny side up. Flatten dough with hands and cover with the second piece of paper, with the shiny side down.

5. Use a rolling pin to roll it to a thickness of ¼ to 18 inch. peel off the top paper from the dough. Gently and then lay the dough on top of the paper on a broiler pan or cookie sheet.

6. Bake per side for about 15 minutes. Remove from oven, and flip the sheet of dough carefully. Remove the oven paper gently.

7. Bake for 15 to 25 minutes more or until very dry. Remove from the oven and set aside.

8. Once cool, cut into 1" squares with a large kitchen knife. serve or store for up to 3 days in an airtight container.

Nutritional Information Per Serving:

Calories: 254, Net Carbs: 1.5g, Fats: 15.5g, Protein: 9.2g, Fiber: 15.6g

Three Cheese Bacon Tomato Frittata

Preparation Time: 10 minutes

Cook Time: 35 minutes

Servings: 8

Ingredients:

6 Slices of bacon, cut into bite size pieces

1 cup Cherry tomatoes, sliced

10 Eggs

1/2 Cup cheddar cheese, shredded

1/4 Cup heavy cream

1/4 Cup parmesan cheese

1/4 Cup feta cheese crumbles

Directions

1. Put the cut bacon on a pan over medium heat and fry until crispy. Add to the pan, the tomatoes and cook 3-4 minutes longer.

2. Whisk the eggs in a large bowl. Add the creams and whisk together thoroughly. Add the cheese to the egg mixture and mix gently with a spatula.

3. Finally, add the egg mixture to the pan and cook 2 more minutes.

4. Place pan inside the oven for 20 to 25 minutes and let it cook at 375 degrees F.

Nutritional Information Per Serving:

Calories: 210, Total Carbs:2.9g, Fats: 16.3g, Protein: 13.8g, Fiber: 0.1g

Avocado and Salmon Low-Carb Breakfast

Preparation Time: 5 minutes

Total Time: 5 minutes

Servings: 1

Ingredients:

1 ripe organic avocado (about 2.5 oz), cut &seeded

2 oz wild caught smoked salmon

1 oz goat cheese, fresh& soft

2 tablespoons organic extra virgin olive oil

The juice of 1 lemon

Pinch of salt

Directions

1. Add the salmon, goat cheese, oil, juice and salt to a small food processor until coarsely chopped.

2. Place the creamy mixture inside the avocado and serve.

Nutritional Information Per Serving:

Calories: 525, Net Carbs: 4g, Fats: 48g, Protein: 19g,

Dairy-Free Egg "Porridge"

Preparation Time: minutes

Total Time: minutes

Servings: 1

Ingredients:

2 organic e eggs

1/3 cup organic coconut milk (without food additives)

1 tablespoon extra virgin coconut oil

Preferred sweetener, to taste

Ground organic cinnamon ,to taste

Directions

1. Add the coconut milk, eggs, and sweetener to a small bowl. Whisk gently.

2. In a medium saucepan, melt the coconut oil over low heat. Add the egg and coconut milk mixture. Cook and mix until thickens..

3. Once it starts to curdle, remove immediately from the heat. Serve sprinkled with cinnamon.

Nutritional Information Per Serving:

Calories: 445, Net Carbs: 4.4g, Fats: 40.5g, Protein: 15.8g,

Keto Scrambled Eggs Recipe

The secret to light, fluffy scrambled eggs is to move them constantly so that they don't take on any color. If desired, you can also add in milk or heavy cream.

Ingredients:

3 Large Eggs

1 tbsp unsalted butter

Coarse salt

Freshly ground pepper

Directions:

1. Beat eggs together with fork. Add butter to a pan, set over low heat and melt. Now add the egg mixture.

2. Use a flexible spatula to pull the eggs gently to the center of the pan. Allow the liquid parts to run out under the perimeter.

3. Cook and move eggs continually with the spatula for 2 to 3 minutes, just until the eggs are set. Add salt and pepper to taste; serve and enjoy.

Nutritional Information Per Serving:

Calories: 318, Net Carbs: 1.8g, Fats: 26.3g, Protein:17.4g,

POULTRY

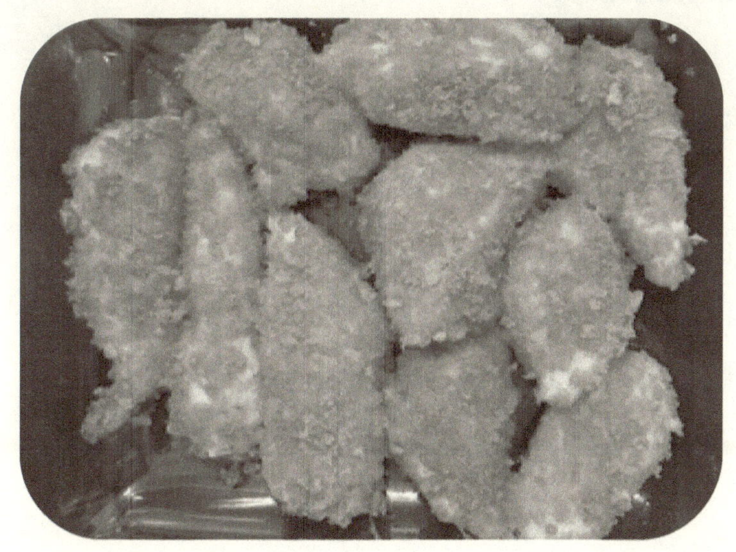

Parmesan Chicken Zoodles With Sun Dried Tomatoes

A recipe that is so good and easy.

Preparation time: 10 minutes

Cooking time: 25 minutes

Servings: 6

Ingredients:

4 ounces of fresh semi-dried tomato strips in oil, diced

3 1/2 ounces of jarred sun dried tomatoes in oil, diced

1 1/2 pounds of chicken thigh fillets, skinless and cut into strips

1 1/4 cup of full fat or reduced fat thickened cream

1 cup of parmesan cheese, shaved

1 tablespoon of butter

4 garlic cloves, peeled and crushed

2 large zucchinis, made into zoodles

Dried basil seasoning

Red chili flakes

Salt

Directions:

1. In a pan, heat the butter over medium high heat, add the chicken and sprinkle salt on it. Cook the chicken until it is well cooked and all its sides turn golden brown.

2. Add the two tomatoes and garlic. Sauté until it becomes fragrant.

3. Reduce the heat, add the parmesan cheese and cream. Simmer the mixture while stirring until the cheese melts totally.

4. Sprinkle the dried basil, chili flakes and salt over it.

5. Add the zoodles, stir and continue to simmer for about 5-8 minutes until the zoodles are soft.

Nutritional Information Per Serving

Calories - 394, Carbohydrates - 9.2g, Fat - 22.6g, Proteins - 35.6g, Fiber - 0.8g

Chicken Dill Salad
Yum and really tasty.

Preparation time: 5 minutes

Cooking time: 0 minutes

Servings: 8

Ingredients:

1 pound of cooked chicken breast, cut into cubes

1/2 cup of chopped celery

1/3 cup of finely chopped onion

3/4 cup of mayonnaise

3 tablespoons of fresh dill

1 tablespoon plus 1 teaspoon of Dijon mustard

Sea salt

Black pepper

Directions:

1. Thoroughly combine all the ingredients together in a large bowl.

2. Eat alone or serve on fresh lettuce leaves.

Nutritional Information Per Serving

Calories - 236, Carbohydrates - 1.5g, Fat - 16.5g, Proteins - 12g, Fiber - 0.25g

Slowcooker Chicken Stew

A simple Asian recipe that will leave you satisfied.

Preparation time: 5 minutes

Cooking time: 2 hours 10 minutes

Servings: 4

Ingredients:

28 ounces of chicken thighs, skinless, boneless and cut into 1-inch pieces

2 cups of chicken stock

1 cup of chopped celery sticks

1 cup of fresh spinach

1/2 cup of chopped onions

1/2 cup of heavy cream

2 medium carrots, peeled and finely chopped

3 cloves of garlic, crushed

1 sprig of fresh rosemary

1/2 teaspoon of dried oregano

¼ of teaspoon dried thyme

1/8 teaspoon of xanthan gum or more

Salt

Pepper

Directions:

1. In a crockpot, add the chicken, stock, onion, carrots, garlic, celery, thyme, oregano and rosemary. Cover and cook for 4 hours on low or 2 hours on high.

2. Season with salt and pepper.

3. Add the heavy cream and spinach, stir.

4. Sprinkle the xanthan gum and add more if needed to achieve your preferred thickness.

5. Keep on whisking and cook for an extra 10 minutes

Nutritional Information Per Serving

Calories - 228, Carbohydrates - 6g, Fat - 11g, Proteins - 23g

Chicken Stir-fry

A simple Asian recipe that will leave you satisfied.

Preparation time: 10 minutes

Cooking time: 12 minutes

Servings: 2

Ingredients:

2 chicken thighs, boneless, skinless and sliced into thin strips

2 heaping cups of bagged broccoli slaw mix

1/2 cup of water

1/2 cup of scallions, chopped

1/4 cup of gluten-free soy sauce

1 tablespoon of sesame oil

1 tablespoon of minced fresh ginger

1 tablespoon of granulated sugar substitute

1 teaspoon of red pepper flakes

1 tsp onion powder

1/2 tsp xanthan gum

1/2 tsp garlic powder

Directions:

1. In a large pan, stir fry the ginger and chicken in oil for 2-3 minutes.

2. Add all the ingredients except the slaw and scallions to the pan. Stir thoroughly and let it simmer for 5 minutes.

3. Add the slaw and scallions, toss to coat and let it simmer for an extra 2 minutes or until al dente.

Nutritional Information Per Serving

Calories - 219, Carbohydrates - 5.5g, Fat - 10g, Proteins - 19g

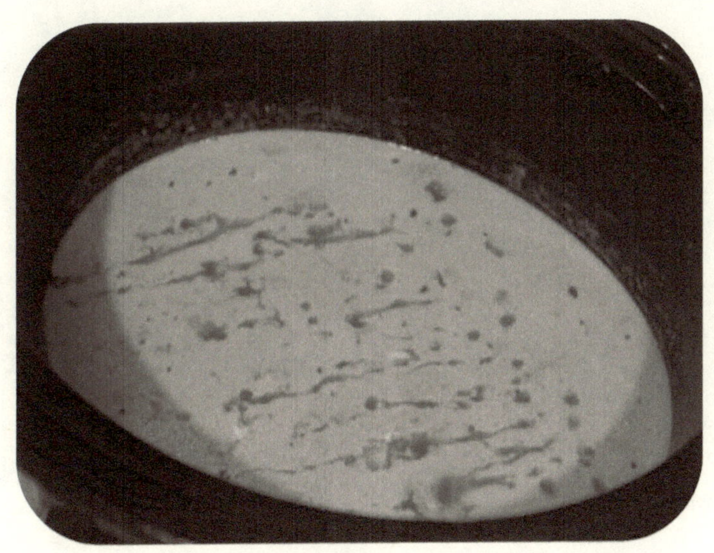

Buffalo Chicken Soup

Buffalo Chicken Soup

A creamy bowl of yum!

Preparation time: 10 minutes

Cooking time: 10 minutes

Servings: 4

Ingredients:

4 ounces of cream cheese

4 cups of chicken broth

2 cups of shredded cooked chicken

1/2 cup of half and half

1/3 cup of red hot sauce

1/4 cup of chopped celery, optional

3 tablespoons of butter

1 tablespoon of blue cheese dressing, optional

Salt &Pepper

Directions:

1. Blend the chicken stock, hot sauce, cream cheese, half and half, and butter in a blender until smooth.

2. Pour into a small saucepan and cook until it is heated. Ensure that it does not boil.

3. To serve, add the chicken, blue cheese and celery. Adjust seasoning if required.

Nutritional Information Per Serving

Calories - 406, Carbohydrates - 5g, Fat - 27g, Proteins - 29g

Curry Chicken Salad

A highly addictive dish.

Preparation time: 10 minutes

Cooking time: 5 minutes

Servings: 2

Ingredients:

2 cups of cooked chicken breast, cut up

1/4 cup of mayo

2 medium celery stalks, sliced finely

2 tablespoons of raw almonds, chopped

1 teaspoon of curry powder

Salt

Directions:

1. Thoroughly mix all the ingredients together in a medium bowl.

2. Serve with a salad or alone.

Nutritional Information Per Serving

Calories - 576, Carbohydrates - 6g, Fat - 29g, Proteins - 55g, Fiber - 2g

Chicken Soup

This classic dish has a warm and inviting flavor.

Preparation time: 15 minutes

Cooking time: 1 hour 40 minutes

Servings: 4

Ingredients:

1 pound of chicken breast, shredded or chopped

4 cups of chicken broth

2 cups of chopped zucchini

1 cup of chopped yellow squash

1 cup of chopped celery

1 cup of chopped onions

1/2 cup of chopped green beans

1 teaspoon of salt

1 teaspoon of basil

Black pepper

Celery salt, optional

Directions:

1. Combine all the ingredients except the celery salt and black pepper in a large pot. Ensure that the broth covers the ingredients. Add water if desired.

2. Boil over high heat. Turn down to a simmer and leave for about 90 minutes while covered.

3. Season with the celery salt and black pepper. Serve.

Nutritional Information Per Serving

Calories - 247, Carbohydrates - 7.75g, Fats - 4.58g, Proteins - 48.58g, Fiber - 3.40g

Turkey Meatballs In Curry Sauce

Whip this dish up for an easy dinner.

Preparation time: 10 minutes

Cooking time: 35 minutes

Servings: 6

Ingredients:

For meatballs:

1.25 pounds of ground turkey

1/3 cup of almond flour

1/4 cup of dessicated coconut

1 egg

1 tablespoon of chopped fresh cilantro

1/2 tablespoon of granulated sugar substitute

1 teaspoon of crushed garlic

1/2 teaspoon of kosher salt

1/4 teaspoon of garlic powder

1/4 teaspoon of red pepper flakes

For sauce:

2 cups of water

6 tablespoons of powdered coconut milk

3 tablespoons of granulated sugar substitute

3 tablespoons of green curry paste

2 tablespoons of fish sauce

1 tablespoon of coconut oil

Directions:

1. In a medium bowl, mix all the meatballs ingredients together and shape into 18 meatballs. Set the balls on a baking sheet lined with parchment paper.

2. Bake the meatballs in the oven for 15 minutes at 375F.

3. In a medium saucepan, cook the curry paste and coconut oil over medium heat for about 2 minutes or until it turns fragrant.

4. Add the remaining sauce ingredients and whisk until it is smooth. Heat for about 10 minutes on low.

5. Add the meatballs to the sauce and simmer for about 5 minutes.

6. Serve.

Nutritional Information Per Serving

Calories - 276, Carbohydrates - 4g, Fat - 22g, Proteins - 16g, Fiber - 0g

Italian Wedding Soup

Quick, simple and incredibly delicious.

Preparation time: 15 minutes

Cooking time: 45 minutes

Servings: 10

Ingredients:

For soup:

6-ounce bag of fresh baby spinach

8 cups of sugar free chicken broth

1 cup of sliced celery

1/4 cup of sliced baby carrots

2 teaspoons of onion powder

2 teaspoons of garlic powder

Salt

Pepper

For meatballs:

1 pound of ground turkey

1 tsp onion powder

1 tsp garlic powder

1 large egg

1/2 teaspoon of dried basil

Directions:

1. Boil the broth in a large pot.

2. Meanwhile, mix all the meatballs ingredients in a medium bowl and shape into meatballs.

3. Drop the balls into the boiling broth gently.

4. Add all the spices and vegetables except the spinach. Cook for about 20-30 minutes until it is well cooked and the carrots are soft.

5. Stir in the spinach quickly and boil the soup for an extra 1-2 minutes.

6. Bring down from heat and leave to cool.

7. Season with salt and pepper.

Nutritional Information Per Serving

Calories - 94, Carbohydrates - 3g, Fat - 5g, Proteins - 10g, Fiber - 1g

Turkey And Bacon Chowder
Luscious and inviting.

Preparation time: 10 minutes

Cooking time: 40 minutes

Servings: 8

Ingredients:

8 ounces of dry aged cherry hardwood smoked bacon, chopped into 1-inch pieces

8 cups of turkey stock

4 cup of cooked turkey meat, chopped or shredded

1/2 cup of heavy whipping cream

1/2 cup of chopped celery

1/2 cup of extra sharp cheddar cheese, shredded

1 tablespoon of fresh thyme leaves

1 large shallot, peeled and chopped

1 teaspoon of dried parsley

1/2 teaspoon of liquid smoke

1 teaspoon of xanthan gum

Salt

Pepper

Directions:

1. In a medium pan, brown the bacon until it is slightly crispy. Remove about 1/4 cup of the bacon, crumble and keep aside.

2. Saute the celery and shallots in the bacon grease for about 5 minutes until soft.

3. Add the cheddar cheese, stock and whipping cream. Whisk until it melts and majorly smooth.

4. Add the liquid smoke, turkey and parsley carefully. Simmer for about 20 minutes.

5. Whisk in the xanthan gum and cook for an extra 5 minutes or until it thickens a bit.

6. Add the thyme, salt and pepper.

7. Garnish with the reserved bacon and fresh thyme leaves

Nutritional Information Per Serving

Calories - 328, Carbohydrates - 6g, Fat - 19g, Proteins - 29g

BEEF

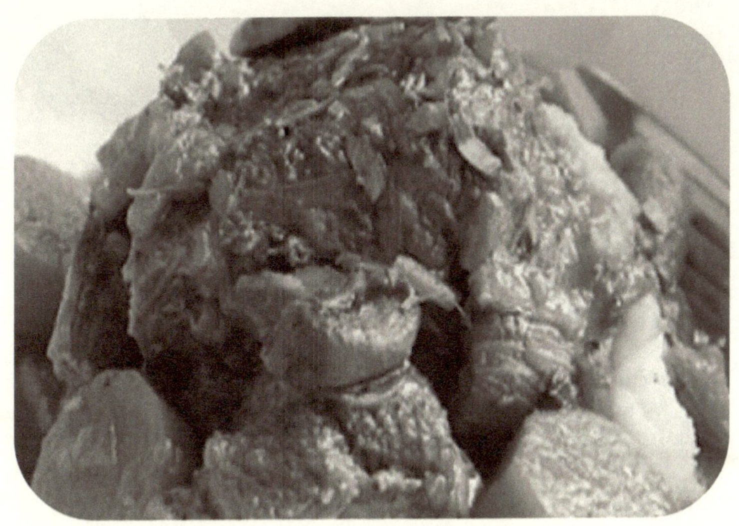

Beef Chili

Absolutely easy and filling!

Preparation time: 3 minutes

Cooking time: 10 minutes

Servings: 4

Ingredients:

1 pound of lean ground beef

1/2 cup of prepared salsa

1 teaspoon of ground coriander

1 teaspoon of ground cumin

1/2 teaspoon of garlic powder

1/2 teaspoon of ground cayenne, optional

Salt and

Pepper

Directions:

1. Mix the beef and spices in a medium saucepan.

2. Add the salsa when the beef is well cooked. Leave to simmer for 5 minutes.

Nutritional Information Per Serving

Calories - 229, Carbohydrates - 2.25g, Fat - 9g, Proteins - 33g

Beef Stroganoff Soup

Settle down to a bowl of this on cold winter nights.

Preparation time: 30 minutes

Cooking time: 6 hours

Servings: 12

Ingredients:

32 ounces of beef stock

10 ounces of cremini mushrooms, sliced thinly

1 1/2 pounds of steak, sliced thinly

1 cup of sour cream

1 cup of heavy cream

3 tables of butter

3 tablespoons of minced garlic

2 tablespoons of chopped Italian flat leaf parsley

2 tablespoons of beef bouillon granules

2 tablespoons of dijon mustard

1 medium onion, chopped

1 ½ teaspoon of garlic powder

1 ½ teaspoon of onion powder

1 teaspoon of dried oregano

1 teaspoon of sea salt

Directions:

1. Preheat your crockpot on high.

2. Add the mushrooms and beef stock to the crockpot. Cover.

3. In a large skillet, sauté the garlic and onions in butter over medium heat until tender and translucent. Add this to the crockpot.

4. Sear both sides of the steak for about 1-2 minutes in the same skillet.

5. Add the steak and the remaining ingredients to the crockpot.

6. Cook for 6 hours on high.

Nutritional Information Per Serving

Calories - 293, Carbohydrates - 4.5g, Fat - 19g, Proteins - 20g

Keto Big Mac Casserole

Preparation time: 20 minutes

Cooking time: 40 minutes

Servings: 6

Ingredients:

2 pounds of ground beef

2 cups of shredded sharp cheddar cheese, packed and divided

1 cup of shredded mozzarella cheese

1 cup of Russian Dressing, divided

1 cup of dill pickle slices

2 garlic cloves, crushed

1 large head of romaine lettuce, chopped

2 tablespoons of sesame seeds, toasted

2 tablespoons of onion flakes, minced

1 tablespoon of Worcestershire sauce

Sea salt

Ground pepper

Directions:

1. Preheat oven to 350F.

2. Brown the beef, garlic, onion flakes, sea salt, Worcestershire sauce and pepper in a large pan over medium heat. Discard the extra grease and put the beef mixture in a casserole dish.

3. Add the mozzarella, 1 cup of cheddar cheese and 3/4 cup of the dill pickles to the beef mixture and thoroughly combine.

4. Flatten the mixture into a compact and even layer. Add the remaining pickles as toppings.

5. Sprinkle the remaining cheddar cheese and sprinkle the sesame seeds on top.

6. Bake for 20 minutes. Increase oven to high broil and cook for an extra 5 minutes.

7. Serve on a bed of lettuce and drizzle the remaining Russian dressing on top.

Nutritional Information Per Serving

Calories - 556, Carbohydrates - 5.8g, Fat - 51g, Proteins - 45g, Fiber - 3g

Slow Cooker Cabbage Roll Soup

Preparation time: 20 minutes

Cooking time: 3 hours

Servings: 9

Ingredients:

16 ounces of marinara sauce

2 pounds of ground beef

5 cups of beef broth

2 cups of cauliflower rice

1/2 cup of shallots, chopped

1/2 cup of onion, chopped

2 tablespoons of extra virgin olive oil

1 large cabbage, sliced

2 cloves of garlic

1 teaspoon of dried parsley

1 teaspoon of pepper

1 teaspoon of salt

1/2 teaspoon of dried oregano

Directions:

1. In a skillet, heat the garlic and oil over medium heat.

2. Sauté the shallots and onions until soft.

3. Add the beef and brown it until it is no longer pink.

4. Add the oregano, parsley, pepper and salt.

5. Add the cauliflower rice and stir until it is well coated.

6. Put the beef mixture into your slow cooker alongside the broth and cabbage. Stir.

7. Cook for 6 hours on low or 3 hours on high.

Nutritional Information Per Serving

Calories -312, Carbohydrates - 9.8g, Fat - 15.2g, Proteins - 31.1g, Fiber - 2.8g

Meatloaf Cupcakes

Warning: you might eat them all at one sitting!

Preparation time: 10 minutes

Cooking time: 30 minutes

Servings: 12

Ingredient:

1 1/2 pounds of minced or ground beef

1 cup of cheese, shredded or grated

2 eggs

1 onion

Salt

Pepper

Directions:

1. Combine the beef, eggs, onion, salt and pepper together.

2. Season with your preferred flavorings and seasonings.

3. Combine everything with your hands and put a small handful of the mixture in muffin tins. Gently press, but not too hard so they don't from turn into meatballs.

4. Top with the cheese.

5. Bake at 350F.

Nutritional Information Per Serving

Calories - 221, Carbohydrates - 1g, Fat - 17.2g, Proteins - 15.2g, Fiber - 0.4g

Keto Greek Stuffed Mushrooms
Seriously delicious!

Preparation time: 15 minutes

Cooking time: 10 minutes

Servings: 12

Ingredients:

For mushrooms

12 mushrooms

11 ounces of minced or ground beef

2 garlic cloves

A handful of fresh basil

Salt

Pepper

For toppings:

12 slices of haloumi

Fresh basil leaves

6 sundried tomatoes

Directions:

1. In a pan, sauté the garlic in oil for 1 minute.

2. Add the meat and stir until is well cooked.

3. Stir in the basil, salt and pepper.

4. Wash or peel the mushrooms to prepare it.

5. Set a tomato on each of the mushrooms.

6. Evenly divide the lamb among the mushrooms and place on a greased baking sheet.

7. Set a basil leaf on top of the mushroom and top with a haloumi piece.

8. Cook in the oven for 10 minutes or until the haloumi is warm and the mushrooms are cooked.

Nutritional Information Per Serving

Calories - 111, Carbohydrates - 1.9g, Fat - 7.7g, Proteins - 8.4g, Fiber - 0.4g

Lamb Burgers

Made with all the flavors of Greek cuisine.

Preparation time: 15 minutes

Cooking time: 5 minutes

Servings: 6

Ingredients:

1 pound of ground beef

1 pound of ground lamb

2 tablespoons of fresh rosemary, chopped

2 garlic cloves, minced

1 teaspoon of dried oregano

1 teaspoon of dried thyme

1 teaspoon of salt

1/2 teaspoon of pepper

Directions:

1. Tear the beef and lamb into small pieces and add to a medium bowl. Use your hands to gently mix them together.

2. Add the rosemary, garlic and the other dry ingredients to the meat. Combine thoroughly with a hand mixer and shape into 6 balls. Flatten the 6 balls into patties.

3. Fry or grill the patties to your taste.

Nutritional Information Per Serving

Calories - 528, Carbohydrates - 5g, Fat - 45g, Proteins - 25g, Fiber - 1g

Lasagna Meatballs

Definitely a winner!

Preparation time: 10 minutes

Cooking time: 45 minutes

Servings: 8

Ingredients:

For Meatballs:

1 pound of hot or sweet Italian sausage

1 pound of ground chuck

1/4 cup of parmesan cheese, grated

1/3 cup almond flour

1 tablespoon of dried parsley

2 eggs

1 teaspoon of kosher salt

1/2 teaspoon of onion powder

1/2 teaspoon of garlic powder

1/4 teaspoon of red pepper flakes

1/4 teaspoon of dried oregano

For Casserole:

2 cups of keto marinara

1 1/2 cups of shredded whole milk mozzarella cheese

1 cup of whole milk ricotta cheese

Directions:

1. Get a baking sheet and line it with parchment paper.

2. In a medium bowl, mix all the meatballs ingredients together and shape into meatballs. Place on the baking sheet.

3. Bake for 15 minutes at 375F.

4. Arrange the meatballs in a single layer in a casserole dish and pour half of the marinara sauce over it.

5. Using teaspoons, drop the cheese over the casserole evenly. Pour the remaining marinara sauce over it and sprinkle the mozzarella on top.

6. Bake at 375F for about 30 minutes. Allow to cool for 5 minutes and then serve.

Nutritional Information Per Serving

Calories - 494, Carbohydrates - 4g, Fat - 39g, Proteins - 31g

Salisbury Steak

Prepare this American classic with ingredients from your pantry.

Preparation time: 12 minutes

Cooking time: 30 minutes

Servings: 6

Ingredients:

For the steaks:

2 pounds of ground chuck

1/4 cup of beef broth

3/4 cup of almond flour

1 tablespoon of chopped fresh parsley

1 tablespoon of Worcestershire sauce

1 tablespoon of dried onion flakes

1/2 teaspoon of garlic powder

1 1/2 teaspoon of kosher salt

1/2 teaspoon of ground black pepper

For The Sauce:

2 cups of button mushrooms, sliced

1 cup of yellow onions, sliced

1/2 cup of beef broth

1/4 cup of sour cream

2 tablespoons of bacon grease

2 tablespoons of butter

1/2 teaspoon of Worcestershire sauce

Salt

Pepper

Directions:

1. In a medium bowl, thoroughly combine all the steak ingredients and shape into 1-inch oval patties. Set the patties on a cookie sheet.

2. Bake for 18 minutes at 375F.

3. In a large pan, melt the bacon grease and butter.

4. Sauté the mushrooms for 2 minutes on each side until golden brown.

5. Sauté the onions over medium heat for 5 minutes.

6. Add the Worcestershire sauce and broth, cook and stir for 2 minutes.

7. Stir in the sour cream and remove from heat.

8. Season with salt and pepper.

9. Serve the sauce over warm steaks and garnish with parsley if desired.

Nutritional Information Per Serving

Calories - 457, Carbohydrates - 5g, Fat - 34g, Proteins - 32g

Crockpot Chili

Made with no beans but still delicious!

Preparation time: 30 minutes

Cooking time: 8 hours

Servings: 2-4

Ingredients:

2 1/2 pounds of ground beef

1 14.5-ounce can of tomatoes and green chilies

1 14.5-ounce can of stewed tomatoes with Mexican seasoning

1 6-ounce can of tomato paste

1/4 cup of pickled jalapeno slices

4 tablespoons of crushed garlic

4 tablespoons of chili powder

2 tablespoons of Worcestershire sauce or Coconut Aminos

2 tablespoons of cumin, mounded

3 large celery ribs, chopped

1 medium red onion, diced and divided

2 teaspoon of sea salt

1 tsp of oregano

1 tsp onion powder

1 tsp garlic powder

1 tsp black pepper

1 bay leaf

1/2 teaspoon of cayenne

Directions:

1. Preheat crockpot on low.

2. Brown the beef, 2 tablespoons of garlic, half of the onions, salt and pepper in a large pan over medium high heat. Drain excess fats once the beef is browned.

3. Put in a crockpot and add the other ingredients.

4. Cover and cook for 6-8 hours on low.

Nutritional Information Per Serving

Calories - 137, Carbohydrates - 4.7g, Fat - 5g, Proteins - 16g

PORK

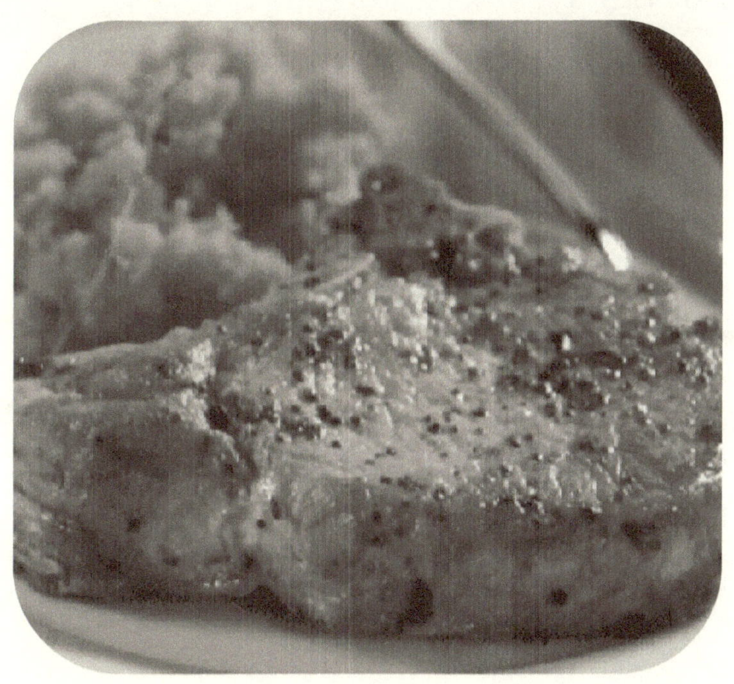

Creamed Lemon Mustard Pork Loin

High in fat and perfect for keto.

Preparation time: 15 minutes

Cooking time: 20 minutes

Servings: 2

Ingredients:

For pork loins:

4 pork loins

1 tablespoon of pink Himalayan sea salt

1 tsp of paprika

1 tsp black pepper

1 tsp thyme

For Mustard Sauce:

1/2 cup chicken broth

1/4 cup heavy cream

1 tablespoon of mustard

1 teaspoon of apple cider vinegar

1/2 lemon, juiced

Directions:

1. Use a paper towel to pat the pork dry and season with the rest of the pork loins ingredients.

2. Sear the pork for about 2-3 minutes per side in a large skillet over high heat. Set aside.

3. Add the heavy cream, broth and vinegar to the skillet. Allow it simmer.

4. Add the mustard and lemon juice. Stir to mix.

5. Add the pork to the sauce and flip it to coat.

6. Cook the pork for about 10 minutes while the lid is slightly kept open.

Nutritional Information Per Serving

Calories - 326, Carbohydrates - 1g, Fat - 30g, Proteins - 46g

Asian Pork Chops
Flavorful, sweet and delicious.

Preparation time: 20 minutes

Cooking time: 4 minutes

Servings: 2

Ingredients:

4 pork chops, boneless

1 tablespoon of almond flour

1 tablespoon of fish sauce

1/2 tablespoon of sambal chili paste

1/2 tablespoon of sugar free ketchup

4 garlic cloves, cut in halves

1 medium star anise

1 lemongrass stalk, peeled and chopped

1 1/2 teaspoon of soy sauce

1 teaspoon of sesame oil

1/2 teaspoon of peppercorns

1/2 teaspoon of five spice

Directions:

1. Wrap a rolling pin in wax paper, place the pork chops on a flat surface and pound to 1/2-inch thick with the rolling pan.

2. Blend the star anise and peppercorns in a blender to a fine powder. Add the garlic and lemongrass to the blender, process until it forms a puree.

3. Add the soy sauce, fish sauce, five- spice and sesame oil. Combine thoroughly.

4. Set the pork chops on a tray, add the blended mixture and coat the pork. Cover and let it marinate for 1-2 hours at room temperature.

5. Coat the pork with almond flour lightly and heat a pan to high.

6. Add the pork to the pan and sear both sides for about 2 minutes per side until it forms a golden crust.

7. Cut each of the pork into strips on a chopping board.

8. Stir the ketchup and sambal chili paste together to make a sauce.

Nutritional Information Per Serving

Calories - 272, Carbohydrates - 6g, Fat - 9.5g, Proteins - 34g

Roasted Pork Shoulder

Succulent, moist and meaty!

Preparation time: 10 minutes

Cooking time: 4 hours 20 minutes

Servings: 12

Ingredients:

8-10 pounds of pork shoulder

For the spice rub:

2 tablespoons of kosher salt

2 tablespoons of garlic powder

1 tablespoon of ground cumin

1 tablespoon of ground black pepper

1 tablespoon of onion powder

1 tablespoon of dried oregano

Directions:

1. In a small bowl, mix all the spice ingredients together.

2. Pat the spice rub all over the pork with your hands. Set it in a large pan with its skin side facing up.

3. Roast for 20 minutes in a preheated oven at 500F.

3. Turn down the heat to 300F and roast each pound for an extra 30 minutes.

4. Remove and allow it rest for 30 minutes.

5. Shred, adjust seasoning and serve.

Nutritional Information Per Serving

Calories - 275, Carbohydrates - 0g, Fat - 15g, Proteins - 33g

Bacon And Onion Smothered Pork Chops
The whole family will love this!

Preparation time: 15 minutes

Cooking time: 40 minutes

Servings: 4

Ingredients:

4 bone-in pork chops, 1-inch thick

6 bacon slices, chopped

1/2 cup of chicken broth

1/4 cup of heavy cream

2 small onions, sliced thinly

1/4 teaspoon of salt

1/4 teaspoon of pepper

Salt

Pepper

Directions:

1. Cook the bacon slices until crispy in a large pan over medium heat. Transfer to a bowl with a slotted spoon and leave the grease.

2. Sauté the onions in the bacon grease and sprinkle with salt and pepper. Cook and stir for 15-20 minutes until the onions are golden brown and soft. Transfer to the bowl containing the bacon.

3. Sprinkle the pork with salt and pepper and increase the heat to medium high.

4. Brown the pork in the pan for 3 minutes on first side. Flip the pork, reduce heat to medium and cook the second side for 7-10 minutes. Transfer to a dish with foil.

5. Add the cream and broth to the pan. Allow to simmer for 2-3 minutes until it thickens. Add the bacon and onions to pan, stir.

6. Add the bacon mixture as toppings on the pork chops.

Nutritional Information Per Serving

Calories - 352, Carbohydrates - 6.30g, Fat - 18.23g, Proteins - 36.98g, Fiber - 1.02g

Slow Cooker Pulled Pork
A contender for the best low carb meal you have ever had.

Preparation time: 5 minutes

Cooking time: 6 hours

Servings: 4

Ingredients:

3 Pounds of Pork Shoulder, boneless

1/2 cup of water

2 teaspoons of garlic powder

2 teaspoons onion powder

2 teaspoons of salt

1 teaspoon of ground allspice

1 teaspoon of paprika

1 teaspoon of mustard powder

1 teaspoon of black pepper

1 teaspoon of celery salt

Directions:

1. Put the pork in your slow cooker.

2. Mix all the spices together in a small bowl and rub it on both sides of the pork.

3. Add water, cover and cook on low for 10 hours or on high for 6 hours.

4. Shred the meat into pieces, till it falls apart. Serve.

Nutritional Information Per Serving

Calories - 265, Carbohydrates - 1g, Fat - 16g, Proteins - 20g

Chinese Pulled Pork

Dump all the ingredients in your crockpot and be on your way.

Preparation time: 10 minutes

Cooking time: 8 hours

Servings: 6

Ingredients:

2 pounds of pork

1 cup of chicken broth

4 tablespoons of sugar free tomato sauce

4 tablespoons of soy sauce

2 tablespoons of garlic paste

1 tablespoon of tomato paste

2 teaspoons of ginger paste

1 teaspoon of smoked paprika

5 drops of liquid sweetener

Directions:

1. Put the pork in a crockpot.

2. In a bowl, mix the other ingredients and pour over the pork.

3. Cover and cook for 7 hours on low.

4. Use a fork to stir the sauce and shred the pork. Cook for an additional 30-60 minutes until the sauce becomes thick.

Nutritional Information Per Serving

Calories - 459, Carbohydrates - 3g, Fat - 35g, Proteins - 30g, Fiber - 0g

Grilled Pork Chop With Pico De Gallo

Unbelievably simple to make!

Preparation time: 10 minutes

Cooking time: 5 minutes

Servings: 1

Ingredients:

For Pork Chop:

1 pork chop

1 tablespoon of extra virgin olive oil

1/4 teaspoon of ground cumin

1/4 teaspoon granulated garlic

Kosher salt

Freshly ground black pepper

For Pico de Gallo:

4-5 grape tomatoes, cut into 6-8 pieces each

1/2 ounce of chopped red onion

1/2 jalapeno chile pepper, diced with seeds

2 tablespoons of chopped cilantro

1 tablespoon of extra virgin olive oil

1 lime wedge, squeezed over combined veggies, rind and pith discarded

Kosher salt

Fresh ground black pepper

Directions:

1. In a bowl, mix all the pico de gallo ingredients together. Keep aside.

2. Preheat grill for 5 minutes.

3. Season both sides of the pork with spices and drizzle oil over it.

4. Place on the grill and cook for 2 minutes on each side.

5. Remove from grill, add the pico de gallo as toppings and serve.

Nutritional Information Per Serving

Calories - 507, Carbohydrates - 8g, Fat - 42g, Proteins - 25g, Fiber - 2g

Keto Marinated Pork Chops

Prepare in bulk and enjoy lunch for a week.

Preparation time: 10 minutes

Cooking time: 60 minutes

Servings: 10

Ingredients:

18 pork chops

½ cup of splenda

½ cup of apple cider vinegar

4 tablespoons of soy sauce

½ teaspoon of ginger

½ teaspoon of pepper

Directions:

1. Process all the ingredients except the chops in a food processor.

2. Put the chops in a greased pan and pour the processed marinade over it.

3. Cook at 350F for 60 minutes. Flip it once at 30 minutes.

4. Chop the meat into bite sized portions and serve.

Nutritional Information Per Serving

Calories - 323, Carbohydrates - 1g, Fat - 14g, Proteins - 46g, Fiber - 0g

Slow Cooker Balsamic Pork Roast

Juicy, tender and delicious!

Preparation time: 10 minutes

Cooking time: 4 hours

Servings: 8

Ingredients:

2 pound of pork shoulder roast, boneless

1/3 cup of balsamic vinegar

1/3 cup of vegetable or chicken broth

1 tablespoon of honey

1 tablespoon of Worcestershire sauce

1/2 teaspoon of garlic powder

½ teaspoon of red pepper flakes

Kosher salt

Directions:

1. Season the pork with red pepper flakes, garlic and salt. Put in a crockpot.

2. In a bowl, combine the Worcestershire sauce, broth and vinegar. Pour this mixture over the pork.

3. Drizzle the honey over the pork and cook on high for 4 hours or on low for 6-8 hours.

4. Use tongs to transfer the pork to a platter and lightly shred with two forks.

Nutritional Information Per Serving

Calories - 214, Carbohydrates - 4g, Fat - 12g, Proteins - 21g, Fiber - 0g

Tomato And Pork Soup

A hearty meal like no other.

Preparation time: 10 minutes

Cooking time: 4 hours 15 minutes

Servings: 8

Ingredients:

2 pounds of country pork ribs, boneless and cut into 1 inch pieces

2 cups of cauliflower rice, finely chopped

2 cups of chopped fresh tomatoes

1 cup of chicken stock

1 cup of water

1/2 cup of dry white wine

1/2 cup of chopped onion

2 tablespoons of chopped fresh oregano

1 tablespoon of olive oil

1 tablespoon of garlic, chopped

Salt

Pepper

Directions:

1. Generously season the pork with salt and pepper.

2. In a heavy saucepan, heat the oil and brown the pork on all sides or until it turns golden.

3. Add the garlic and onion, cook for additional 2 minutes.

4. Add the stock, white wine, tomatoes and water. Stir and allow to boil.

5. Pour into a crockpot and cook for 4 hours on high.

6. Stir in the oregano and cauliflower in the final 15-20 minutes of cooking.

Nutritional Information Per Serving

Calories - 326, Carbohydrates - 3g, Fat - 22g, Proteins - 21g

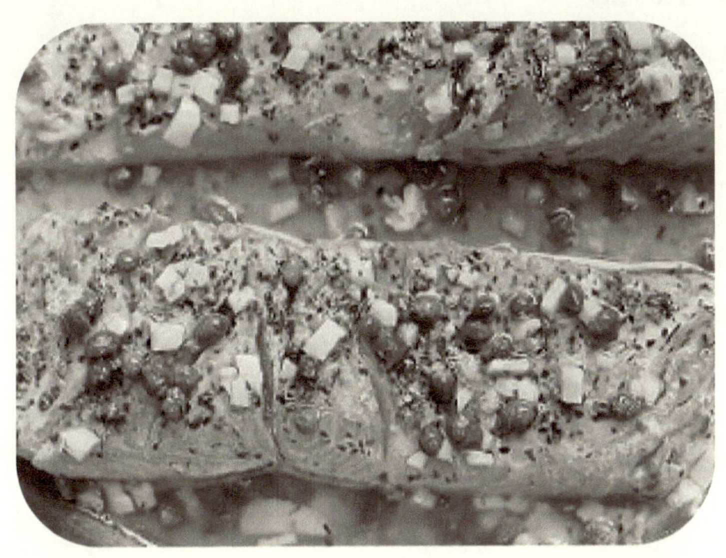

Fish Cakes
Packed with tons of flavor.

Preparation time: 2 minutes

Cooking time: 8 minutes

Servings: 1

Ingredients:

For the Fish Cakes:

1 tin of tuna in springwater

1 tablespoon of mayonnaise

1 egg

4 tablespoons of almond flour

1 tablespoon of olive oil

2 teaspoons of Thai Red Curry Paste

For the Lime Mayonnaise:

1/2 tablespoon of lime juice

2 tablespoons of mayonnaise

1 teaspoon of coriander paste

Directions:

1. In a small bowl, thoroughly mix all the fish cake ingredients together.

2. Heat oil in a large pan over medium heat. Scoop the fish mixture with a tablespoon into the pan, flatten it slightly to form cakes.

3. Cook for 2-4 minutes per side until crisp.

4. Mix the lime mayonnaise ingredients in a bowl and serve over the hot fish cakes.

Nutritional Information Per Serving

Calories - 644, Carbohydrates - 8g, Fat - 64g, Proteins - 12g, Fiber - 3g

Keto Bacon Wrapped Scallops
An elegant dish prepared in few minutes.

Preparation time: 5 minutes

Cooking time: 5 minutes

Servings: 4

Ingredients:

12 scallops

12 toothpicks

12 thin slices of microwaveable bacon

1 tablespoon of oil

Salt

Pepper

Directions:

1. Heat the oil in a pan over high heat.

2. Use the bacon slices to wrap each scallop. Secure it with a toothpick and season with salt and pepper.

3. Cook each side for 2 1/2 minutes.

Nutritional Information Per Serving

Brazilian Shrimp Stew

A traditional Brazilian dish that is super mouthwatering.

Preparation time: 10 minutes

Cooking time: 20 minutes

Servings: 6

Ingredients:

1 1/2 pounds of raw shrimp, peeled & deveined

1 14-ounce can of diced tomatoes with chili

1 cup of coconut milk

1/4 cup of chopped fresh cilantro

1/4 cup of olive oil

1/4 cup of chopped roasted red pepper

1/4 cup of chopped onion

2 tablespoons of fresh lime juice

2 tablespoons of sriracha hot sauce

1 clove garlic, minced

Salt

Pepper

Directions:

1. In a medium saucepan, heat the oil and sauté the onions for some minutes until it turns translucent.

2. Add the peppers and garlic, cook for some extra minutes.

3. Add the shrimp, tomatoes and cilantro. Gently simmer until the shrimp turns opaque.

4. Add the sriracha and coconut milk, cook until it is well heated. Ensure that it does not boil.

5. Add the lime juice, salt and pepper.

6. Garnish with fresh parsley and serve.

Nutritional Information Per Serving

Calories - 294, Carbohydrates - 5g, Fat - 19g, Proteins - 24g, Fiber - 0g

Lobster Bisque

A dish to comfort you when the weather gets cold.

Preparation time: 20 minutes

Cooking time: 1 hour 20 minutes

Servings: 4

Ingredients:

24 ounces of lobster chunks

1 quart of seafood broth

1 ounce of brandy

2 cups of white wine

1 cup of heavy cream

1/2 cup of tomato paste

1 tablespoon of olive oil

1 tablespoon of salt

1 tablespoon of fresh lemon juice

4 garlic cloves, finely chopped

4 celery stalks, finely chopped

3 bay leaves

2 carrots, finely chopped

1/2 red onion, finely chopped

1 teaspoon of xanthan gum

1 teaspoon of peppercorns

1 teaspoon of thyme

1 teaspoon paprika

Parsley

Directions:

1. In a pot, Sauté the onion in oil until it turns fragrant. Add the garlic and cook until the pot becomes crusty at the bottom and a bit black.

2. Use the wine to deglaze the pot before adding the carrot and celery.

3. Add the brandy, tomato paste and brandy. Stir to mix.

4. Add the spices and summer for 60 minutes.

5. Remove the bay leaves on the soup is cooked.

6. Add the heavy cream and bring to a simmer again.

7. Gradually add the xanthan gum while stirring.

8. Blend the soup in a blender until it is creamy. Pour into a bowl and add the lobster. Stir to mix.

9. Garnish with parsley, chives, green onion and lemon juice.

Nutritional Information Per Serving

Calories - 220, Carbohydrates - 8g, Fat - 15g, Proteins - 12g

Coconut Shrimp
Absolutely fancy!

Preparation time: 10 minutes

Cooking time: 6 minutes

Servings: 2

Ingredients:

For the shrimp:

12 large shrimp

6 tablespoons of mayonnaise

3 tablespoons of unsweetened coconut milk

2 tablespoons of flaked coconut

2 tablespoons of coconut, shredded

1 egg yolk

For the dip:

4 tablespoons of mayo

1 teaspoon of unsweetened lime juice

2 teaspoons of chili garlic sauce

Directions:

1. Thaw the shrimp and dry it.

2. In a bowl, combine the remaining shrimp ingredients and coat the shrimp with it.

3. Cook the shrimp in the fryer until it turns golden brown.

4. On another bowl, combine the dip ingredients and serve with the shrimp.

Nutritional Information Per Serving

Calories - 6, Carbohydrates - 7g, Fat - 69g , Proteins - 11g, Fiber - 3g

Fish Chowder

This amazing chowder will leave you craving for more.

Preparation time: 10 minutes

Cooking time: 30 minutes

Servings: 6

Ingredients:

4 bacon slices, chopped

1 pound of fresh white fish, chopped

3 cups of daikon radish

2 1/2 cups of chicken stock

2 cups of heavy cream

1 tablespoon of butter

1/2 teaspoon of dried thyme

1 medium onion, diced

Salt

Pepper

Directions:

1. Cook the bacon in a large saucepan over medium heat until crisp. Using a slotted spoon, transfer to a plate lined with paper towels.

2. Cook the radish and onions in the bacon fat for about 10 minutes until the onions becomes soft.

3. Pour in the stock and leave to simmer for 10 minutes. Add the pepper, thyme and salt to season.

4. Add the fish and heavy cream. Simmer for an extra 4 minutes until the fish is well cooked.

5. Top with the butter and serve.

Nutritional Information Per Serving

Calories - 364, Carbohydrates - 4.7g, Fat - 16g, Proteins - 24g, Fiber - 1.3g

Fish Curry
Bursting with delicious flavors!

Preparation time: 5 minutes

Cooking time: 20 minutes

Servings: 6

Ingredients:

2.2 pounds of white fish, cubed

1.1 pounds of spinach, washed and sliced

1 2/3 cups of water

1 2/3 cups of coconut cream

2 tablespoons of curry paste

Directions:

1. In a large saucepan, heat oil and fry the curry paste for 2-3 minutes over moderate heat.

2. Add the water and coconut cream, allow to boil.

3. Add the fish carefully, turn down the heat and allow to simmer for 10-15 minutes.

4. Add the spinach and cook for an additional 3-4 minutes or until it wilts.

5. Serve!

Nutritional Information Per Serving

Calories - 314, Carbohydrates - 5.8g, Fat - 18.5g, Proteins - 33.4g, Fiber - 2.2g

Seafood Soup

Celebrate your love for seafood with this delightful dish.

Preparation time: 25 minutes

Cooking time: 1 hour

Servings: 6

Ingredients:

For the soup:

10 ounces of wild cod

8 ounces of shrimp, peeled

8 ounces of calamari, cut into 1/2-inch pieces

8 ounces of mushrooms, chopped

1 quart of seafood broth

2 cups of water

1.5 cup of tomato sauce

1/2 cup of coconut cream

1/4 cup of coconut oil

4 garlic cloves, minced

4 celery stalks, chopped

4 green onion stalks, chopped

3 medium carrots, chopped

1 medium onion, chopped

1 lemon, juiced

1 lime, juiced

For the spices:

3 whole bay leaves

1 tablespoon of salt

2 teaspoons of oregano

2 teaspoons of red pepper flakes

2 teaspoons of basil

2 teaspoons of pepper

1 teaspoon of dill

1 teaspoon of thyme

Fresh parsley

Directions:

1. In a soup pot, heat 2 tablespoons of oil over medium heat and sauté the garlic and onions until fragrant.

2. Add the celery and carrots. Cook the veggies until soft.

3. Pour in the water, broth and tomato sauce. Bring to a boil and turn down the heat to a simmer and leave it to simmer for about 30 minutes.

4. Put the shrimp and calamari in a bowl containing lemon juice and leave to sit for a while.

5. After the pot has been simmering for about 30 minutes, add the chopped mushrooms and coconut cream.

6. Add the cod after about 10 minutes and leave it to cook for an extra 10 minutes.

7. Break the cod into little pieces with a wooden spoon.

8. Add the shrimp and cook for about 3 minutes.

9. Then add the calamari to the pot and cook for an additional 2 minutes.

10. Remove from heat, discard the bay leaves and add the lime juice.

11. Serve with parsley and green onion.

Nutritional Information Per Serving

Calorie s - 284, Carbohydrates - 9g, Fat - 14g, Proteins - 27g, Fiber - 0g

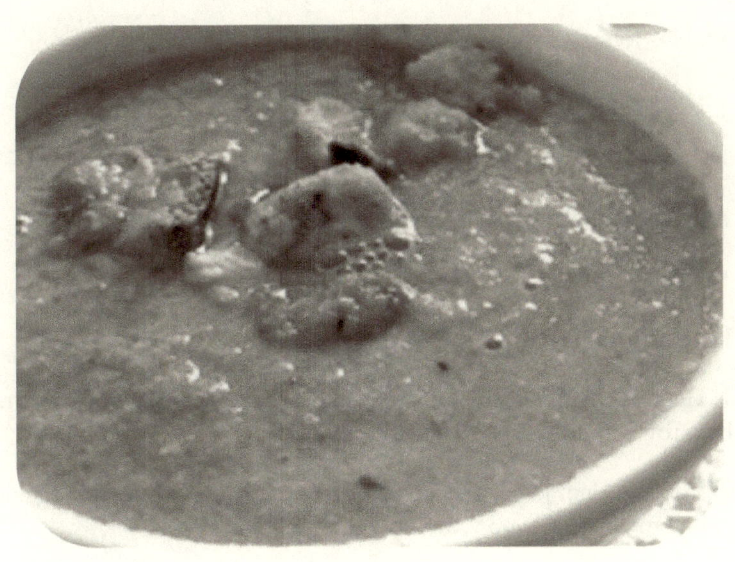

Lobster Bisque Soup

Seafood Chowder
Leaves you feeling full and satisfied!

Preparation time: 20 minutes

Cooking time: 10 minutes

Servings: 6

Ingredients:

12 cherry tomatoes

10 ounces of clams

4 ounces of canned blue crab

3 medium celery stalks

1/2 pound of shrimp

1 1/2 cups of chicken broth

4 tablespoons of clam juice

4 tablespoons of shallots, chopped

2 tablespoons of light olive oil

1/2 teaspoon of garlic

1/8 teaspoon of black pepper

1/8 teaspoon of Italian seasoning

Directions:

1. Heat oil in a medium pot and sauté the shallot and garlic over medium heat for 2 minutes until it turns translucent.

2. Add the clam juice, tomatoes, broth, celery, Italian seasoning and pepper. Allow to simmer for 3 minutes.

3. Add the crab, clams and shrimp to the pot. Cook for 5 minutes until the shrimp are pink and firm.

Nutritional Information Per Serving

Calories - 163, Carbohydrates - 5.1g, Fat - 7g, Proteins - 20.2g, Fiber - 0.9g

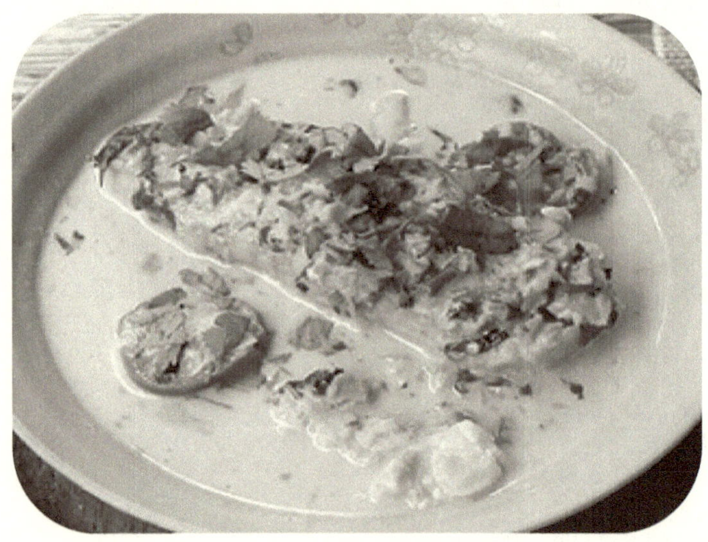

Fish Curry

Thai Seafood Soup

A quality Thai cuisine

Preparation time: 20 minutes

Cooking time: 35 minutes

Servings: 8

Ingredients:

2 pounds of white fish filet, scales and bones removed, cut into 1-inch pieces

2 cans of water chestnuts

4 cups of bone broth

1 cup of coconut milk

1/4 cup of olive oil

2 tablespoons of fish sauce

2 tablespoons of wasabi powder

2 teaspoons of salt

4 cloves of garlic, chopped

4 baby bok choy

3 carrots, chopped

3 lemons, juiced

2 bay leaves

1 large vidalia onion, chopped

1 bunch of cilantro, chopped

Directions:

1. Heat 2 tablespoons of fat in a large pot over medium heat and sauté the onions, garlic, carrots and bay leaves for about 8 minutes until soft. Stir occasionally.

2. Meanwhile, cut, wash and tear the bok choy. Peel some lemon rinds and add to the pot.

3. Stir in the fish until all the pieces are seared.

4. Add the fish sauce, wasabi powder and salt. Stir together.

5. Pour in the broth and allow it boil for 10 minutes.

6. Stir in the water chestnuts and bok choy and let it simmer for 10 minutes.

7. Stir in the lemon juice and adjust seasoning if needed.

8. Garnish with the cilantro, drizzle the rest of the olive oil on it.

9. Serve.

Nutritional Information Per Serving

Calories - 315, Carbohydrates - 8g, Fat - 17g, Proteins - 28g, Fiber - 0g

VEGETABLES

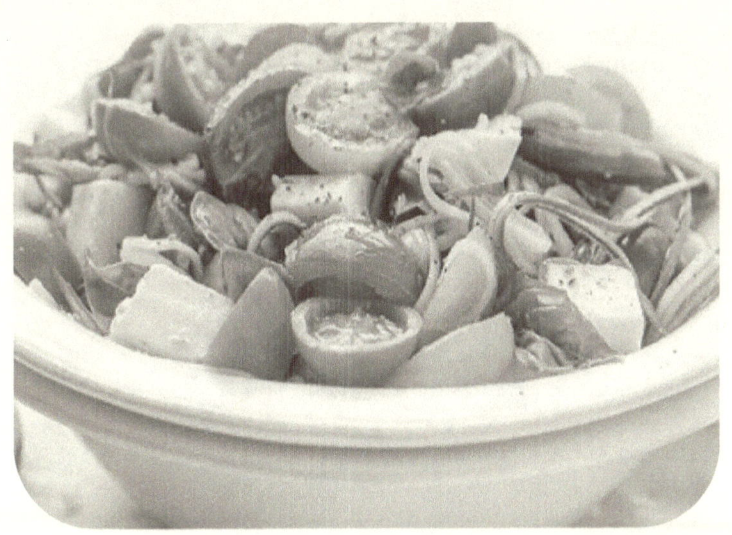

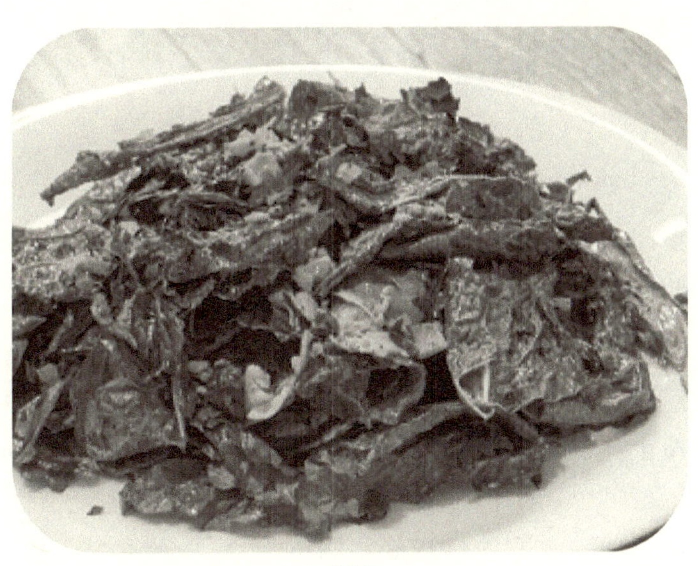

Fried Cauliflower Rice

Has healthy fats needed by the body.

Preparation time: 15 minutes

Cooking time: 15 minutes

Servings: 2

Ingredients:

1 ounce of bell pepper, chopped

1 bacon slice, chopped

1/2 cup of spring onions, sliced

1/3 cup of frozen peas

3 tablespoons of peanut oil

3 tablespoons of wheat free soy sauce

2 eggs

1/2 whole cauliflower, grated

1 teaspoon of sesame oil

Directions:

1. In a bowl, beat the eggs lightly.

2. In a pan, heat half of the peanut oil over low heat and scramble the eggs. Transfer to a plate and keep aside.

3. Lightly brown the bacon in the pan while stirring constantly to prevent burning.

4. Add the cauliflower while constantly stirring. Add the remaining peanut oil.

5. Add in the spring onions and peas while constantly stirring.

6. Stir in the soy sauce and sesame oil.

7. Add the scrambled eggs, stir quickly and serve.

Nutritional Information Per Serving

Calories - 295, Carbohydrates - 9g, Fat - 27g, Proteins - 7g, Fiber - 3g

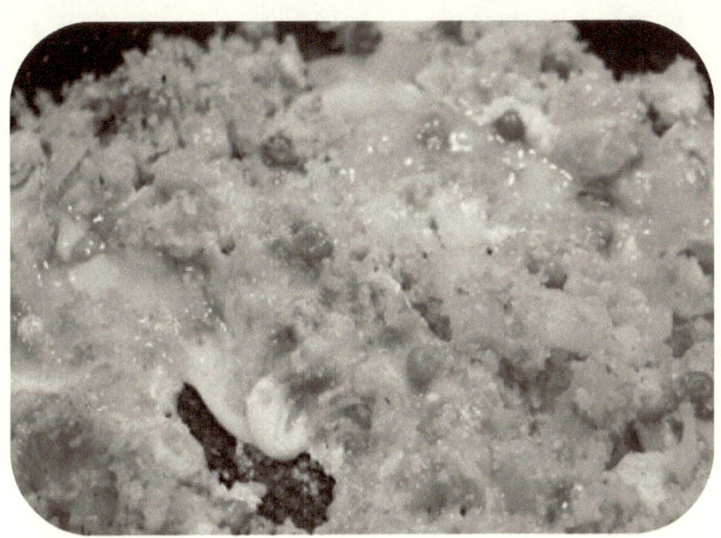

Leek Broccoli Soup

Creamy and packed with flavors!

Preparation time: 5 minutes

Cooking time: 15 minutes

Servings: 3

Ingredients:

1 pound of broccoli, cut into even-sized florets

3 ounces of salted butter

2 1/2 cups of chicken broth

1/2 cup of heavy cream

1 tablespoon of chopped parsley

1 garlic clove

1 medium-sized leek, white parts only, roughly chopped

1 teaspoon of salt

1 teaspoon of pepper

Directions:

1. In a large saucepan, sauté the garlic and leeks in butter over low heat until they start to turn translucent.

2. Add the heavy cream and broccoli to the pan.

3. Pour in the broth and stir to combine. Simmer for 8 minutes on low - medium heat.

4. Blend the soup carefully with a stick blender. Ensure that there are no lumps.

5. Add the parsley, salt and pepper.

Nutritional Information Per Serving

Calories - 402, Carbohydrates - 9g, Fat - 38g, Proteins - 6g, Fiber - 6g

Asian Broccoli Salad
A crispy salad drenched in the flavors of Asia.

Preparation time: 5 minutes

Cooking time: 10 minutes

Servings: 8

Ingredients:

12-ounce bag of broccoli slaw

2 tablespoons of coconut oil

1/2 cup of full fat plain goat milk yogurt

1 tablespoon of coconut aminos

1/2 tablespoon of sesame seeds

1/2 teaspoon of salt

1 teaspoon of grated fresh ginger

Cilantro, optional

Directions:

1. In a large pan, heat the oil over medium heat and cook the broccoli for 7 minutes while covered.

2. Remove the cover, add the ginger, coconut aminos, salt and pepper. Stir to combine.

3. Bring down pan for from heat, add yogurt and top with the sesame seeds.

4. Garnish with the cilantro and serve.

Nutritional Information Per Serving

Calories - 62, Carbohydrates - 3.62g, Fat - 4.28g, Proteins - 1.8g, Fiber - 0g

Cream Of Mushroom Soup
A creamy and absolutely tasty dish.

Preparation time: 10 minutes

Cooking time: 30 minutes

Servings: 2

Ingredients:

2 cups of cauliflower florets

1 1/2 cups of white mushrooms, chopped

1 1/2 cups of unsweetened almond milk

1/2 teaspoon of extra virgin olive oil

1 tsp onion powder

1/4 teaspoon of Himalayan rock salt

Freshly ground pepper

1/2 yellow onion, chopped

Directions:

1. Boil the cauliflower, onion powder, almond milk, salt and pepper in a small covered pan over medium heat.

2. Turn down the heat to low and simmer, until the cauliflower is soft, for 7-8 minutes.

3. Puree the soup in a blender, food processor or immersion blender.

4. In the meantime, in a medium saucepan, saute the onions and mushrooms in oil for about 8 minutes until the onions are translucent and start to brown.

5. Add the cauliflower purée to the pan and leave to boil.

6. Cover the pan and let it simmer for 10 minutes until it thickens.

Nutritional Information Per Serving

Calories - 95, Carbohydrates - 7.9g, Fat - 4g, Proteins - 4.9g, Fiber - 4.4g

Creamy Spinach

Savor this creamy and thick dish on busy weeknights.

Preparation time: 10 minutes

Cooking time: 15 minutes

Servings: 3

Ingredients:

10 ounces of frozen spinach

3 ounces of cream cheese

3 tablespoons of Parmesan cheese

2 tablespoons of sour cream

1/4 teaspoon of onion powder

1/4 teaspoon of garlic powder

Salt

Pepper

Directions:

1. Thaw the spinach in the microwave for about 6-7 minutes until warmed through.

2. Heat a pan over medium high heat, add the spinach and boil off some of the water from it. Season the spinach and stir.

3. Stir in the cream cheese until it melts.

4. Add the sour cream and mix. Reduce the heat to low.

5. Add the Parmesan and stir until the dish thickens.

Nutritional Information Per Serving

Calories - 165, Carbohydrates - 3.63g, Fat - 13.22g, Proteins - 7.34g,

Keto Cabbage Slaw

A nutrient-dense vegetable meal.

Preparation time: 10 minutes

Cooking time: 0 minutes

Servings: 4

Ingredients:

For salad:

2 cups of green cabbage, shredded

2 cups of red cabbage, shredded

1/4 cup of carrots, shredded

2 tablespoons of sesame seeds

2 scallions, thinly sliced

For dressing:

1 tablespoon of sesame oil

1 tablespoon of rice wine vinegar

1 tablespoon of tamari

1/2 teaspoon of garlic, crushed

1/2 teaspoon of ginger, grated

Directions:

1. Combine all the dressing ingredients and set aside.

2. Combine the scallions, cabbages and carrots in a large bowl and toss with the dressing.

3. Garnish with a sprinkling of the sesame seeds.

Nutritional Information Per Serving

Calories - 84, Carbohydrates - 4.5g, Fat - 5.8g, Proteins - 2.6g, Fiber - 2.3g

Beet Stew

Put your stash of beets to work in this amazing recipe.

Preparation time:

Cooking time:

Servings: 4-6

Ingredients:

3 cups of vegetable stock

2 cups of green cabbage, shredded

1 cup of beets, shredded

1/2 cup of carrots, shredded

2 tablespoons of olive oil

1-2 tablespoons of lemon juice

1/2 teaspoon of garlic powder

1/2 teaspoon of onion powder

Salt

Pepper

Directions:

1. In a pot, sauté the cabbage, beets and carrots in olive oil over medium low heat.

2. Add the stock and seasonings. Simmer until the vegetables are cooked through and soft.

Nutritional Information Per Serving

Calories - 95, Carbohydrates - 6g, Fat - 7g, Proteins - 1g, Fiber - 2g

Cauliflower Mash
Much better than mashed potatoes.

Preparation time: 10 minutes

Cooking time: 10 minutes

Servings: 6

Ingredients:

4 ounces of sour cream

1 pound of cauliflower florets

1 cup of Cheddar cheese, grated

3 tablespoons of butter

2 tablespoons of water

2 tablespoons of snipped chives

2 bacon slices, cooked and crumbled

1/4 teaspoon of garlic powder

Salt

Pepper

Directions:

1. Add the cauliflower florets and water to a microwaveable bowl, cover the bowl with cling film and microwave for 5-8 minutes until soft and

thoroughly cooked. Drain excess water, uncover and allow to sit for 1-2 minutes.

2. Process the cauliflower in a food processor until fluffy.

3. Add the sour cream, butter and garlic powder to the food processor. Blend until it resembles mashed potatoes.

4. Pour into a bowl and add some part of the chives.

5. Add half of the Cheddar and combine with your hand. Add salt and pepper to season.

6. Top the cauliflower with the bacon, remaining Cheddar cheese and chives.

7. Melt the cheese in the microwave for some minutes.

8. Serve.

Nutritional Information Per Serving

Calories - 199, Carbohydrates - 5g, Fat - 17g, Proteins - 8g, Fiber - 2g

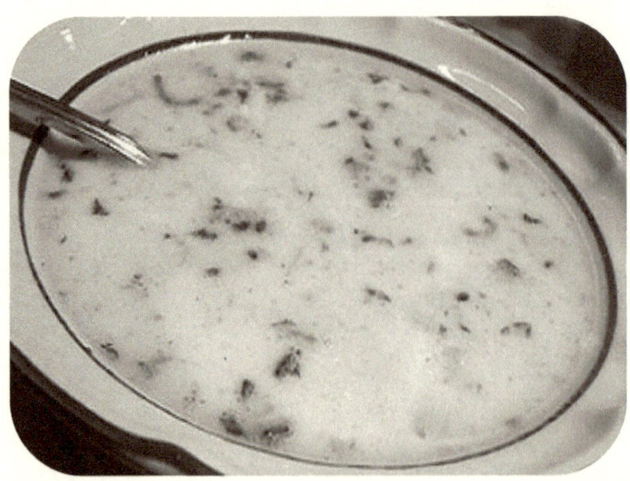

Broccoli Soup With Cheese

Cauliflower Soup

Preparation time: 5 minutes

Cooking time: 20 minutes

Servings: 4

Ingredients:

1 pound of cauliflower, cut into even sized pieces

2 ounces of salted butter

1 cup of heavy cream

2 teaspoons of salt

1 teaspoon of ground white pepper

1/2 teaspoon of ground nutmeg

Directions:

1. Put the cauliflower into a pan, add the cream and fill it with water until the cauliflower tips are just above the water. Bring to a boil.

2. Turn down to a simmer for 10 minutes until it is very soft and can be broken easily with a spoon.

3. Add the nutmeg, salt and pepper.

4. Use a stick blender to blend until smooth.

Nutritional Information Per Serving

Calories - 337, Carbohydrates - 8g, Fat - 34g, Proteins - 4g, Fiber - 3g

Creamy Leeks

Fast and simple to prepare.

Preparation time: 5 minutes

Cooking time: 10 minutes

Servings: 4

Ingredients:

2 large leeks, sliced

2 tablespoons of cream cheese

2 tablespoons of butter

2 garlic cloves, minced

Black pepper

Directions:

1. In a large pan sauté the garlic in the butter.

2. Add the leeks to the pan. Cook and stir until soft.

3. Bring down the pan from heat and stir in the pepper and cream cheese.

4. Serve.

Nutritional Information Per Serving

Calories - 105, Carbohydrates - 7.2g, Fat - 8.4g, Proteins - 1.2g, Fiber - 0.8g

SIDES

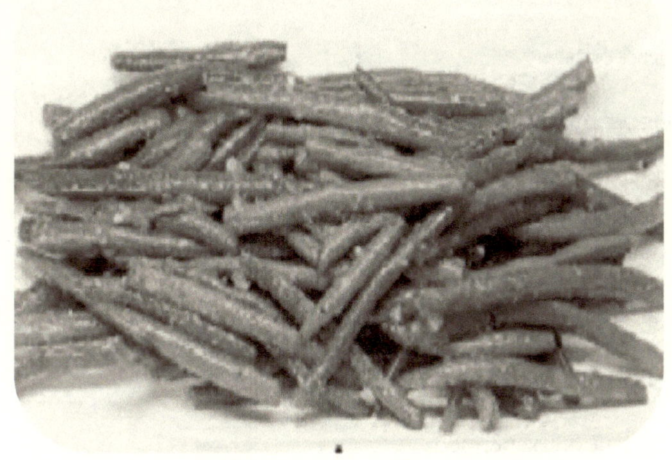

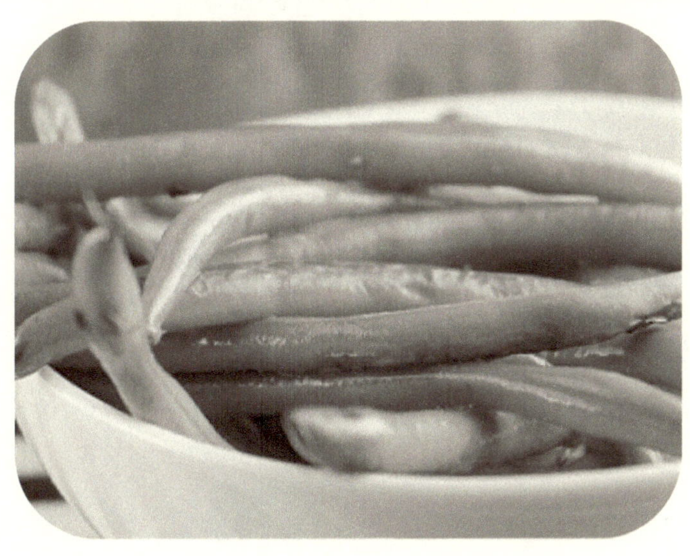

Broccoli, Chives and Sour Cream Mash

A unique addition to any barbecue.

Preparation time: 5 minutes

Cooking time: 10 minutes

Servings: 4

Ingredients:

3 ounces of sour cream

1 ounce of butter

1 pound of broccoli, cut into even sized florets

2 tablespoons of finely chopped chives

1/2 teaspoon of salt

1/2 teaspoon of pepper

Directions:

1. Boil a large pot of water, add the broccoli and cook for 3-5 minutes until soft. Drain and return to the pot.

2. Add the sour cream, butter, salt and pepper to the pot.

3. Using a stick blender, blend the mixture until there are no lumps.

4. Add the chives, stir and adjust seasoning.

Nutritional Information Per Serving

Calories - 134, Carbohydrates - 9g, Fat - 10g, Proteins - 4g, Fiber - 5g

Zucchini Tots

An ingenious way of getting your kids to eat their vegetables.

Preparation time: 5 minutes

Cooking time: 20 minutes

Servings: 6

Ingredients:

2 cups of zucchini, grated

1/2 cup of parmesan cheese

1/2 cup of cheddar cheese, shredded

1/4 cup of onion, chopped

2 large eggs

1 teaspoon of garlic powder

Directions:

1. Preheat oven to 400F.

2. With a tea or paper towel, squeeze out excess water from the zucchini.

3. In a large bowl, thoroughly combine the zucchini with the remaining ingredients.

4. Grease a muffin tin with coconut oil and fill it with the mixture.

5. Bake for 15-20 minutes or until the top is golden brown.

Nutritional Information Per Serving

Calories - 82, Carbohydrates - 2g, Fat - 3.4g, Proteins - 4g, Fiber - 0.3g

Keto Grilled Tomatoes With Apricot Jam

A great side for any grilled meat.

Preparation time: 10 minutes

Cooking time: 25 minutes

Servings: 6

Ingredients:

3 1/2 ounces of gouga cheese, grated

1 1/2 ounces of watercress

6 medium tomatoes, halved

1 tablespoon of olive oil

3 teaspoons of no-sugar apricot jam

2 teaspoons of dried oregano

Salt

Pepper

Directions:

1. Preheat oven to 360F.

2. Grease a baking tray lightly and place the tomato halves on it. Spread some jam on each of the tomato halves and sprinkle the oregano on top.

3. Top the tomatoes with the grated cheese and cook for 25 minutes or until the cheese turns golden.

4. Garnish each tomato with watercress and drizzle with olive oil to serve.

Nutritional Information Per Serving

Calories - 107, Carbohydrates - 4.4g, Fat - 7.2g, Proteins - 5.5g

Keto Hollandiase Asparagus

Add a touch of fanciness to your meals with this really easy dish.

Preparation time: 15 minutes

Cooking time: 25 minutes

Servings: 4

Ingredients:

40 spears of asparagus

1/4 cup of butter, cut into cubes

2 egg yolks

1 tablespoon of fresh lemon juice

A dash of cayenne

Salt

Pepper

Directions:

1. Grease a baking sheet, spread out the asparagus on it and roast for about 10-15 minutes.

2. In a bowl, beat the egg yolks until they are slightly paler in color. Whisk in the lemon juice and heat in a small pan over low flame.

3. Stir until the egg yolks become thick then begin to add 1-2 cubes of butter at a time. Whisk until the sauce is well mixed. Season with cayenne, salt and pepper.

4. Drizzle the sauce over the asparagus and serve.

Nutritional Information Per Serving

Calories - 150, Carbohydrates - 2g, Fat - 13g, Proteins - 3g

Grilled Portobello Mushrooms

Enjoy this meal that's filled with lots of exotic herbs.

Preparation time: 15 minutes

Cooking time: 10 minutes

Servings: 4

Ingredients:

12 ounces of portobello mushroom, sliced about 1/2" thick

2 tablespoons of balsamic vinegar

2 tablespoons of olive oil

1/2 teaspoon of basil

1/2 teaspoon of rosemary

1/2 teaspoon of tarragon

1/2 teaspoon of thyme

Pink Himalayan sea salt

Directions:

1. Preheat your grill.

2. Whisk the oil, herbs and vinegar together. With a pastry or silicone brush, brush the mixture on both sides of the mushrooms.

3. Set the mushrooms on the grill and heat for about 3-5 minutes on each side.

4. Sprinkle the sea salt on top and serve.

Nutritional Information Per Serving

Calories - 84, Carbohydrates - 2g, Fat - 7g, Proteins - 3g

Summer Slaw With Chia Papaya Dressing

A staple for all your summer gatherings.

Preparation time: 10 minutes

Cooking time: 0 minutes

Servings: 8

Ingredients:

For dressing:

1 cup of papaya, peeled and chunked

2 tablespoons of white vinegar

2 tablespoons of light olive oil or avocado oil

1 tablespoon of ginger, minced

A pinch of salt

For slaw:

4 cups of shredded white cabbage

2 cups of mango, sliced into strips

2 cups of shredded red cabbage

1/2 cup of pineapple, sliced into strips

1/4 cup of fresh basil, cut into thin ribbons

1 tablespoon of chia seeds, optional

Directions:

1. In a medium bowl, combine all the slaw ingredients.

2. Blend all the dressing ingredients in a blender or magic bullet until smooth.

3. Drizzle the dressing over the slaw and toss to coat well.

4. Serve the slaw chilled.

Nutritional Information Per Serving

Calories - 90, Carbohydrates - 10g, Fat - 4g, Proteins - 2g

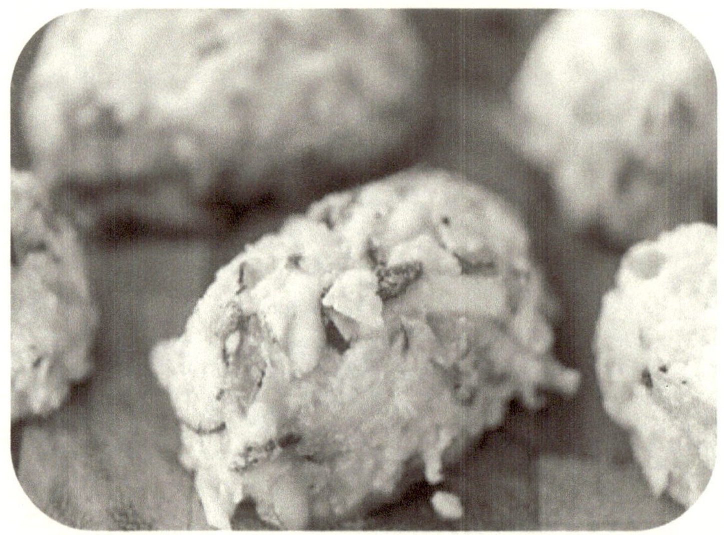

Zucchini Tots

Roasted Turnip, Apple And Celery Puree

Pair this puree with your roasted meat.

Preparation time: 15 minutes

Cooking time: 45 minutes

Servings: 12

Ingredients:

4 cups of turnips, peeled and chopped

1/3 cup of chopped onion

4 cups of chopped celery root

1 cup of unsweetened almond milk

1 cup of granny Smith apples, peeled, cored, and chopped

1/4 cup of heavy cream

1/4 cup of butter

2 tablespoons of olive oil

1 teaspoon of prepared horseradish

Salt

Pepper

Directions:

1. In a large bowl, mix the celery root, onion, apples, olive oil, turnips, salt and pepper. Toss until it is well coated and spread out the mixture on a cookie sheet.

2. Roast for 45 minutes at 325F or until it is tender and golden brown.

3. Blend the veggies in a food processor or blender along with the butter, almond milk, horseradish and heavy cream until smooth.

4. Adjust seasoning and serve hot.

Nutritional Information Per Serving

Calories - 114, Carbohydrates - 7g, Fat - 8g, Proteins - 2g

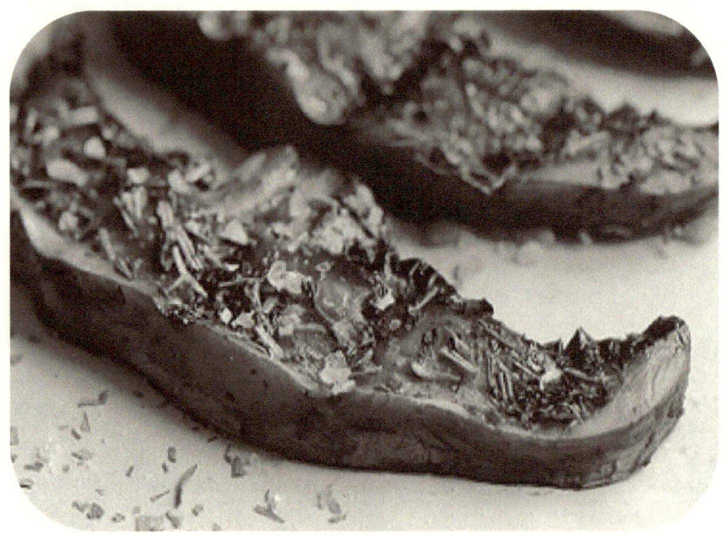

Portobello Mushroom

Broccoli Slaw

A low carb side dish with amazing flavors.

Preparation time: 7 minutes

Cooking time: 0 minutes

Servings: 6

Ingredients:

4 cups of bagged broccoli slaw

1/3 cup of no-sugar mayonnaise

2 tablespoons of granulated sugar substitute

1 1/2 tablespoons of apple cider vinegar

1 tablespoon of Dijon mustard

1 tablespoon of extra virgin olive oil

1 teaspoon of celery seeds

1/2 teaspoon of kosher salt

1/4 teaspoon of black pepper

Directions:

1. Whisk together all the ingredients except the broccoli in a large bowl until it is well mixed.

2. Add the broccoli and toss until well coated.

Nutritional Information Per Serving

Calories - 110, Carbohydrates - 2g, Fat - 10g, Proteins - 2g

Ranch Roasted Broccoli

A unique combination of tangy and sweet.

Preparation time: 5 minutes

Cooking time: 40 minutes

Servings: 6

Ingredients:

4 cups of broccoli florets

1/2 cup of shredded sharp cheddar cheese

1/4 cup of ranch dressing

1/4 cup of heavy whipping cream

Kosher salt

Pepper

Directions:

1. Preheat oven to 375F.

2. In a medium bowl, toss all the ingredients together until the broccoli is coated well and spread out in casserole dish.

3. Bake for 30 minutes.

4. Remove from oven and stir.

5. Return to oven and bake for an extra 5-10 minutes.

Nutritional Information Per Serving

Calories - 135, Carbohydrates - 3g, Fat - 11g, Proteins - 4g

Roasted Green Beans

A North African inspired dish.

Preparation time: 5 minutes

Cooking time: 30 minutes

Servings: 6

Ingredients:

6 cups of raw green beans, trimmed

2 tablespoons of olive oil

1 tablespoon of Ras el Hanout seasoning

1 teaspoon of kosher salt

1/2 teaspoon of ground black pepper

Directions:

1. Toss all the ingredients together in a bowl and spread out in a large roasting pan or cookie sheet.

2. Roast for 20 minutes at 400F.

3. Remove and stir.

4. Put in oven and roast for an extra 10 minutes.

5. Serve chilled or warm.

Nutritional Information Per Serving

Calories - 73, Carbohydrates - 4g, Fat - 5g, Proteins - 2g

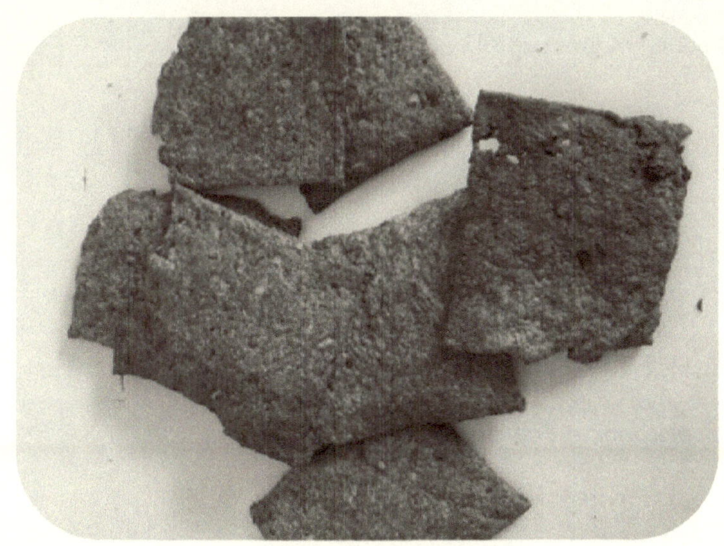

Caprese Meatballs

Crispy and savory!

Preparation time: 15 minutes

Cooking time: 6 minutes

Servings: 4

Ingredients:

1 pound of ground turkey

1/2 cup of whole milk mozzarella, shredded

1/4 cup of almond flour

1 egg

2 tablespoons of fresh basil, chopped

2 tablespoons of olive oil

2 tablespoons of chopped sundried tomatoes

1/2 teaspoon of salt

1/2 teaspoon of garlic powder

1/4 teaspoon of ground black pepper

Directions:

1. In a medium bowl, thoroughly mix all the ingredients except the oil and shape into 16 meatballs.

2. In a large non-stick saute pan, heat the oil and add the meatballs, leaving about 1-inch space between them.

3. Cook each side for about 3 minutes over low or medium heat until well-cooked. Ensure that the cheese does not burn.

Buffalo Chicken Tenders
Moist and cooked to perfection.

Preparation time: 10 minutes

Cooking time: 30 minutes

Servings: 6

Ingredients:

6 ounces of buffalo sauce

1 pound of chicken breast tenders

1 cup of almond flour

1 large egg

1 tbsp heavy whipping cream

Salt

Pepper

Directions:

1. Preheat oven to 350F.

2. Season the chicken with salt and pepper.

3. Generously season the flour with salt and pepper.

4. Whisk the egg and cream together.

5. Dip the chicken in the egg mixture before coating it in the flour mixture. Put the chicken in a baking pan that has been greased lightly.

6. Bake for 30 minutes.

Nutritional Information Per Serving

Calories - 285, Carbohydrates - 3g, Fat - 14.7g, Proteins - 29.3g, Fiber - 3g

Haloumi Cheese Fries

A crunchy cheese stick eaten with any dip.

Preparation time: 5 minutes

Cooking time: 5 minutes

Servings: 4

Ingredients:

2 ounces of tallow

8 ounces of haloumi cheese

A serve of reduced-carb marinara sauce

Directions:

1. Cut the haloumi into the shape of fries that are at least 0.3-inch thick. Leave it on a paper towel to dry.

2. In a nonstick frying pan, add the tallow and set over medium-high heat.

3. Use a pair of tongs to add the pieces of haloumi gently. Cover pan with a splatter guard.

4. Cook each side of the haloumi for about 2 minutes until it is crunchy and golden brown.

5. Serve with the marinara sauce.

Nutritional Information Per Serving

Calories - 200, Carbohydrates - 1g, Fat - 18g, Proteins - 12g, Fiber - 0.3g

Cheesy Bites

The ultimate party appetizer.

Preparation time: 5 minutes

Cooking time: 14 minutes

Servings: 4

Ingredients:

1/2 cup of almond flour

1/2 cup of cheddar cheese, shredded

1/4 cup of mozzarella cheese, shredded

1/4 cup of parmesan cheese, grated

2 eggs

1/4 teaspoon of parsley flakes

1/4 teaspoon of garlic powder

Salt

Pepper

Directions:

1. Preheat oven to 400F.

2. Whisk the eggs, salt and pepper in a bowl.

3. Add the remaining ingredients and stir until it forms a dough.

4. Divide the dough into 8 portions and roll each portion into a ball. Place the balls into a baking sheet lined with parchment paper.

5. Bake for 14 minutes until it is slightly crisp and golden brown.

Nutritional Information Per Serving

Calories - 222, Carbohydrates - 2g, Fat - 17g, Proteins - 15g

Jalapeno Bacon Poppers

Guaranteed to be a hit at your next party.

Preparation time: 5 minutes

Cooking time: 40 minutes

Servings: 16

Ingredients:

6 ounces of ground beef

2 ounces of cream cheese

8 medium-size jalapenos, seeded and halved lengthwise

8 bacon slices, halved lengthwise

Salt

Pepper

Directions:

1. Cook the beef in a pan over medium heat. Add the seasonings and keep aside to cool.

2. Spread the cheese inside each jalapeno half and ensure you do not overfill it so as to leave space for the beef. Top with the beef.

3. Use the bacon to wrap around the jalapeno and place on a baking rack.

4. Bake for 30 minutes at 400F.

Calories - 56.9, Carbohydrates - 0.8g, Fat - 4.6g, Proteins - 3.5g, Fiber - 0.2g

Broccoli Tots

A healthier alternative to tater tots.

Preparation time: 15 minutes

Cooking time: 24 minutes

Servings: 20

Ingredients:

2 cups of raw or frozen broccoli

1/3 cup of Italian breadcrumbs

1/3 cup of cheddar cheese

1/3 cup of panko breadcrumbs

¼ cup of yellow onion, chopped

1 large egg

2 tablespoons of parsley

½ teaspoon of pepper

½ teaspoon of salt

Directions:

1. Preheat oven to 400F.

2. Line a baking sheet with parchment paper or grease with a thin layer of oil. Keep aside.

3. In boiling water, blanch the broccoli for 1 minute. Remove and drench with cold water in order to stop it from cooking. Drain well.

4. Finely chop the broccoli and combine it vigorously with onion, eggs, cheddar, breadcrumbs, salt and pepper.

5. Spoon about 1 1/2 tablespoons of the broccoli mix and press gently into a firm ball between your hands. Form into a tater-tot shape and set on the baking sheet.

6. Bake for 18-24 minutes while turning halfway, until it is golden brown and crisp.

Nutritional Information Per Serving

Calories - 95, Carbohydrates - 9.2g, Fat - 3.6g, Proteins - 5.4g, Fiber - 2g

Pizza Dip

Preparation time: 5 minutes

Cooking time: 25 minutes

Servings: 8

Ingredients:

8 ounces of cream cheese

2 ounces of mozzarella cheese

2 ounces of pepperoni

1/2 cup of sour cream

1/2 cup of tomato sauce

1 teaspoon of oregano

1/2 teaspoon of onion powder

1/4 teaspoon of garlic powder

1/4 teaspoon of red pepper flakes

1/4 teaspoon of salt

1/8 teaspoon of black pepper

Directions:

1. Preheat oven to 350F.

2. In a bowl, mix the sour cream, cream cheese, oregano, onion powder, garlic powder, and red pepper flakes together. Spread the mixture into a 9-inch baking pan's bottom.

3. Add the tomato sauce as toppings and season with salt and pepper.

4. Layer the pepperoni on top and bake for 15 minutes.

5. Remove, layer the mozzarella on top and bake for an extra 10 minutes or until the cheese melts fully.

Nutritional Information Per Serving

Calories - 162, Carbohydrates - 3.75g, Fat - 14g, Proteins - 6g, Fiber - 0.25g

Chia Seed Crackers

Eat alone or enjoy with your favorite dip.

Preparation time: 10 minutes

Cooking time: 40 minutes

Servings: 19

Ingredients:

3 ounces of cheddar cheese, shredded

1 1/4 cup of ice water

1/2 cup of ground chia seeds

2 tablespoons of olive oil

2 tablespoons of psyllium husk powder

1/4 teaspoon of Xanthan gum

1/4 teaspoon of oregano

1/4 teaspoon of garlic powder

1/4 teaspoon of paprika

1/4 teaspoon of onion powder

1/4 teaspoon of salt

1/4 teaspoon of pepper

Directions:

1. Preheat oven to 375F.

2. Combine all the dry ingredients in a bowl and add the olive oil. Mix until it achieves a wet sand texture.

3. Add water and thoroughly mix to form a solid batter.

4. Add the cheese and mix with your hands. Put in a silpat and leave to stand for some minutes.

5. Roll or spread the batter into the silpat size.

6. Bake for 30-35 minutes. Remove and divide into individual crackers.

7. Put back in the oven and broil for 5-7 minutes or until the top of the crackers are crispy.

Nutritional Information Per Serving

Calories - 31, Carbohydrates - 0.1g, Fat - 2.5g, Proteins - 1.3g

Corndog Muffin

Preparation time: 10 minutes

Cooking time: 14 minutes

Servings: 10

Ingredients:

1/2 cup of flaxseed meal

1/2 cup of blanched almond flour

1/3 cup of sour cream

1/4 cup of melted butter

1/4 cup of coconut milk

10 lit'l smokies

1 large egg

3 tablespoons of swerve sweetener

1 tablespoon of psyllium husk powder

1/4 teaspoon of baking powder

1/4 teaspoon of salt

Directions:

1. Preheat oven to 375F.

2. In a bowl, combine all the dry ingredients together. Add the cream, butter, coconut milk and egg to the mixture and combine thoroughly.

3. Grease 20 mini muffin slots and evenly divide the batter between them.

4. Slice the lit'l smokies in half and insert it into each muffin's center.

3. Bake for 12 minutes and then broil for 1-2 minutes until the tops brown lightly.

Nutritional Information Per Serving

Calories - 79, Carbohydrates - 0.7g, Fat - 6.8g, Proteins - 2.4g,

Bacon Jalapeno Fat Bombs

A spicy bomb that is sure to please everyone.

Preparation time: 10 minutes

Cooking time: 5 minutes

Servings: 3

Ingredients:

3 ounces of cream cheese

1 medium-sized jalapeno pepper, seeded and chopped

3 bacon slices

1/2 teaspoon of dried parsley

1/4 teaspoon of garlic powder

1/4 teaspoon of onion powder

Salt

Pepper

Directions:

1. Fry the bacon slices until crispy. Drain on paper towels and keep aside. Reserve the bacon grease.

2. Combine the bacon grease, jalapeno, cream cheese, parsley, garlic powder and onion powder. Season with salt and pepper.

3. Crumble the bacon into a plate. With your hands, roll the cream cheese mixture into balls and then roll the ball into the bacon.

Nutritional Information Per Serving

Calories - 207, Carbohydrates - 1.5g, Fat - 19.3g, Proteins - 4.8g,

DESSERTS

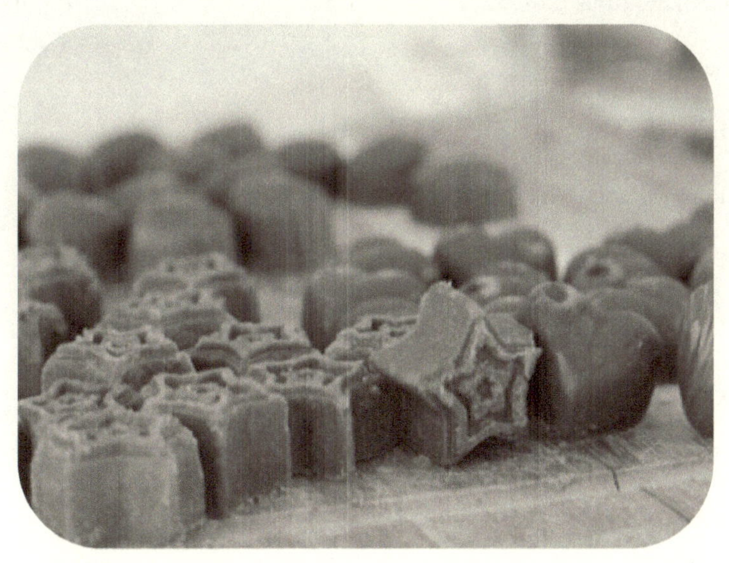

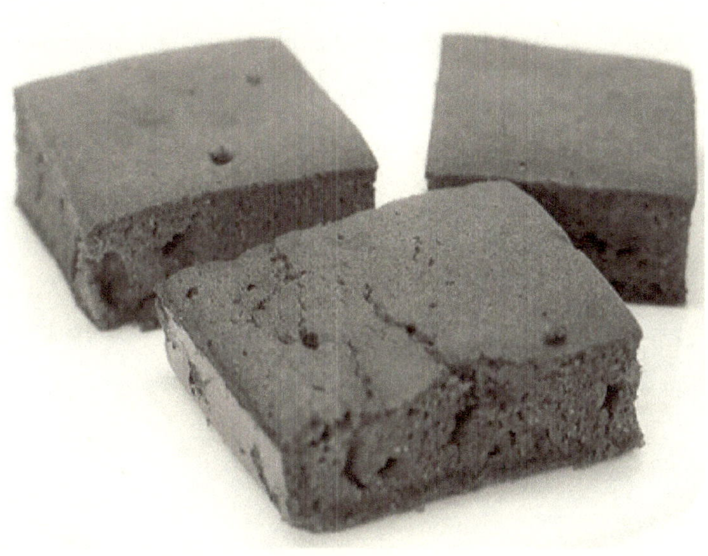

No-Sugar Peanut Butter Fudge

A fantastic guilt-free recipe.

Preparation time: 5 minutes

Cooking time: 0 minutes

Servings: 12

Ingredients:

1 cup of coconut oil

1 cup of unsweetened peanut butter

1/4 cup of unsweetened vanilla almond milk

2 teaspoons vanilla liquid stevia, optional

A pinch of salt, optional

Directions:

1. In a stove set on low heat or microwave, melt the coconut oil and peanut butter slightly.

2. Put in your blender along with the other ingredient and blend until it is well mixed.

3. Line a loaf pan with parchment paper and pour the mixture into it.

4. Keep in refrigerator for about 2 hours until it sets.

Nutritional Information Per Serving

Calories - 287, Carbohydrates - 4g, Fat - 29.7g, Proteins - 5.4g, Fiber - 1.4g

Lemon Cheesecake Mousse

Perfect for times when your body needs a treat.

Preparation time: 10 minutes

Cooking time: 0 minutes

Servings: 5

Ingredients:

8 ounces of cream cheese or mascarpone cheese

1 cup of heavy cream

1/4 cup of lemon juice

1 cup heavy cream

1/2-1 teaspoon of lemon liquid stevia

1/8 teaspoon of salt

Directions:

1. Blend the cheese and lemon juice in a stand mixer until smooth.

2. Add the remaining ingredients and blend together until whipped.

3. If desired, adjust sweetener.

4. Keep refrigerated until it is time to serve.

Nutritional Information Per Serving

Calories - 277, Carbohydrates - 1.7g, Fat - 29.6g, Proteins - 3.7g,

Chocolate Pudding

A delicious pudding that is also dairy-free.

Preparation time: 10 minutes

Cooking time: 2 minutes

Servings: 2

Ingredients:

1 tablespoon of dark cocoa powder

2 tablespoons of sweetener

1 cup of unsweetened coconut milk

1/2 teaspoon of glucomannan powder

Directions:

1. In a microwaveable bowl, pour the coconut milk and add the cocoa powder and sweetener. Whisk the mixture thoroughly.

2. While still whisking, gradually sprinkle the glucomannan powder over it. Whisk thoroughly to remove lumps.

3. Heat the bowl in a microwave for 1 minute 30 seconds or until it is heated but not boiling.

4. Remove and give a final whisk.

5. Cover the bowl and refrigerate for some hours or until the mixture thickens and becomes cold.

Nutritional Information Per Serving

Calories - 81, Carbohydrates - 3.3g, Fat - 6.5g, Proteins - 2.1g

Blueberry Cheesecake Squares

Simply fast to make and incredibly tasty!

Preparation time: 10 minutes

Cooking time: 20 minutes

Servings: 9

Ingredients:

1/2 cup of frozen blueberries

1/2 cup of cream cheese, cubed

1 stick plus 2 tablespoons of melted butter or coconut oil

6 eggs

4 tablespoons of granulated sweetener

2 teaspoons of vanilla

1/2 teaspoon of baking powder

Directions:

1. In a mixing bowl, combine all the ingredients except the blueberries, with a stick blender until smooth.

2. Line an 8-inch baking dish and pour the batter into it.

3. Evenly drop the berries gently throughout the batter.

4. Bake for 20-30 minutes at 320F until the center is cooked.

5. Cool completely before cutting into 9 squares.

Nutritional Information Per Serving

Calories - 220, Carbohydrates - 2.5g, Fat - 21.5g, Proteins - 4.8g, Fiber - 0.4g

Keto Brownies

A yummy dessert that requires no flour.

Preparation time: 10 minutes

Cooking time: 20 minutes

Servings: 12

Ingredients:

4 ounces of softened cream cheese

2/3 cup of unsweetened cocoa

1 1/2 sticks of butter, melted

6 eggs

4 tablespoons of granulated sweetener

2 teaspoons of vanilla

1/2 teaspoon of baking powder

Directions:

1. In a mixing bowl, combine all the ingredients with a stick blender until smooth.

2. Line a baking dish and pour the batter into it.

3. Bake for 20-25 minutes at 350F until the center is cooked.

4. Cut into triangle wedges, squares or rectangle bars.

Nutritional Information Per Serving

Calories - 178, Carbohydrates - 3.5g, Fat - 17g, Proteins - 4.5g, Fiber - 2g

Peanut Butter Chocolate Cake

Amazingly moist and awesome!

Preparation time: 15 minutes

Cooking time: 1 minute

Servings: 1

Ingredients:

2 tablespoons of erythriol or swerve

2 tablespoons of organic unsweetened cocoa powder

1 tablespoon of heavy cream

1 tablespoon of peanut butter

1 large-size pastured egg

1 teaspoon of salted butter

1/2 teaspoon of vanilla extract

1/4 teaspoon of baking powder

Directions:

1. Whisk the erythriol, cocoa powder and baking powder in a small mixing bowl with a fork. Ensure to break up any clumps formed by the baking powder.

2. Whisk the heavy cream, egg and vanilla extract in another bowl. Pour this mixture into the baking powder mixture and combine thoroughly.

3. In a small bowl or ramekin, melt the butter and swirl to coat.

4. Pour the dough into the coated bowl or ramekin and microwave for a minute and 20 seconds.

5. Heat the peanut butter in the microwave to soften it and drizzle over the cake.

Nutritional Information Per Serving

Calories - 246, Carbohydrates - 5g, Fat - 19g, Proteins - 10g

Macaroon Fat Bombs
A small piece is enough to leave you satisfied.

Preparation time: 10 minutes

Cooking time: 15 minutes

Servings: 10

Ingredients:

1/2 cup of coconut, shredded

¼ cup of organic almond flour

2 tablespoons of Swerve

1 tablespoon of coconut oil

1 tablespoon of vanilla extract

3 egg whites

Directions:

1. Combine the flour, swerve and coconut in a bowl until thoroughly mixed.

2. In a small saucepan, melt the oil and add the vanilla to it.

3. Meanwhile, chill a medium-size bowl for mixing the egg whites, in a freezer.

4. Add the melted oil to the flour mixture and combine thoroughly.

5. Whisk the egg whites in the cold medium bowl until it turns foamy and forms stiff peaks.

6. Add the egg whites to the flour mix gently. Try to preserve some of the egg whites' volume and ensure you do not overmix.

7. Scoop the mixture into muffin cups or a cookie sheet.

8. Bake for 8 minutes at 400F or until it is browned on top.

Nutritional Information Per Serving

Calories - 46, Carbohydrates - 0.5g, Fat - 5g, Proteins - 1.8g, Fiber - 0.5g

Coconut Raspberry Bark Fat Bombs
Satiate your sweet tooth cravings.

Preparation time: 25 minutes

Cooking time: 10 minutes

Servings: 12

Ingredients:

1/2 cup of unsweetened coconut, shredded

1/2 cup of freeze dried raspberries

1/2 cup of coconut oil

1/2 cup of coconut butter

1/4 cup of powdered Swerve Sweetener

Directions:

1. Use parchment paper to line an 8 x 8 baking pan.

2. Pulse the raspberries into fine powder in a food processor or coffee grinder. Keep aside.

3. Mix the shredded coconut, butter, swerve and coconut oil in a medium saucepan and cook over medium heat. Stir often until the ingredients melts and are well mixed.

4. Put half of the coconut mix into the baking pan. Add the ground raspberries to the mixture in the pan. Stir thoroughly until mixed.

5. Fold the ground raspberry mix over the top of the coconut mix in the saucepan. Use a knife to swirl the mixture together.

6. To set, refrigerate or freeze. Then break it into chunks.

Nutritional Information Per Serving:

Calories - 234, Carbohydrates - 6.56g, Fat - 23.56g, Proteins - 1.72g, Fiber - 4.11g

Food energy: 234kcal Total fat: 23.56g

Caramel Machiatto Cheesecakes

An elegant dessert to indulge in.

Preparation time: 20 minutes

Cooking time: 15 minutes

Servings: 9

Ingredients:

Cheesecakes:

8 ounces of softened cream cheese

1/3 cup of granulated sugar substitute

3 eggs

3 tablespoons of espresso or cold brew coffee concentrate

2 tablespoons of unsalted butter

1 tablespoon of no sugar caramel flavored syrup

Frosting:

8 ounces of softened mascarpone cheese

3 tablespoons of no sugar caramel flavored syrup

3 tablespoons of softened unsalted butter

2 tablespoons of granulated sugar substitute

Directions:

For cheesecakes:

1. Line a cupcake pan with paper liners or grease 9 silicone cupcake molds.

2. Blend all the cheesecake ingredients in a blender until smooth.

3. Bake for 15 minutes at 350F or until it sets. Freeze for an hour or refrigerate for at least 3 hours.

For frosting:

4. Cream the stevia, syrup and butter until it is fluffy.

5. Add the mascarpone and blend at low speed until it is smooth.

6. Spoon the frosting on the cheesecakes and serve.

Nutritional Information Per Serving

Calories - 286, Carbohydrates - 1g, Fat - 29g, Proteins - 5g

Mocha Mousse

A bite of this decadent recipe will leave you craving for more.

Preparation time: 20 minutes

Cooking time: 0 minutes

Servings: 4

Ingredients:

Cream Cheese Mixture:

8 ounces of softened cream cheese

1/4 cup of unsweetened cocoa powder

1/3 cup of granulated stevia erythriol blend

3 tablespoons of sour cream

2 tablespoons of softened butter

3 teaspoons of instant coffee powder

1 1/2 teaspoons of vanilla extract

Whipped Cream Mixture:

1/2 teaspoon of vanilla extract

1 1/2 teaspoons of granulated stevia erythriol blend

2/3 cup of heavy whipping cream

Directions:

1. Using an electric mixer, combine the sour cream, butter and cream cheese until smooth.

2. Add in the stevia, vanilla extract, coffee powder and cocoa powder. Combine until well mixed. Keep aside.

3. Beat the whipping cream in another bowl until it forms soft peaks. Add the vanilla extract and stevia and combine until it forms stiff peaks.

4. Fold 1/3 of the whipped cream mix into the cheese mix in order to lighten it. Ensure that you do not pop the bubbles.

5. Fold in the rest of the whipped cream mix until it is well mixed.

6. Divide among serving plates, keep in the refrigerator to set.

Nutritional Information Per Serving

Calories - 421.75, Carbohydrates - 6.57g, Fat - 41.94g, Proteins - 6.03g

STAPLES

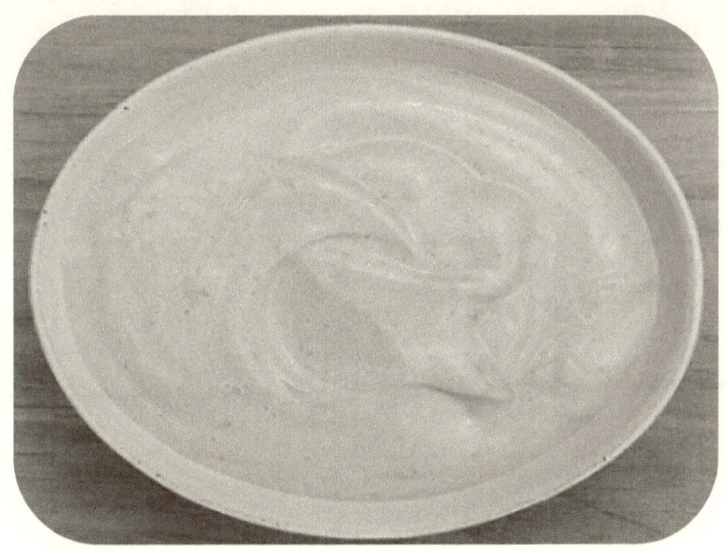

Pesto

An extremely flavorful condiment.

Preparation time: 10 minutes

Cooking time: 0 minutes

Servings: 24

Ingredients:

1 ½ cups of fresh basil

1/3 cup of toasted pine nuts

2/3 cup of olive oil

¾ cup of Parmesan cheese, grated

2 teaspoons of tomato paste

1 teaspoon of crushed garlic

Salt

Pepper

Directions:

1. Blend all the ingredients except the oil in an emulsion blender until smooth.

2. While still blending, add the oil slowly.

3. Store in a mason jar.

Nutritional Information Per Serving

Calories - 79, Carbohydrates - 0.73g, Fat - 8.09g, Proteins - 1.22g

Bone Broth

Amazingly rich!

Preparation time: 45 minutes

Cooking time: 24 hours

Servings: 12

Ingredients:

10 cups of filtered water

3 chicken carcasses

2 tablespoons of apple cider vinegar

2 tablespoons of peppercorns

3 bay leaves

1 lemon

3 teaspoon of turmeric

1 teaspoon of salt

Directions:

1. Preheat the oven to 400F.

2. Put the chicken carcass on a sheet pan, sprinkle with salt and roast for 45 minutes. Transfer them to a crockpot.

3. Add the water, peppercorns, vinegar and bay leaves. Cover and cook for 24-48 hours on low.

4. Cover a large bowl with a fine mesh strainer or sieve and strain the broth. Dispose of the peppercorns, bones and bay leaves. Divide the broth among 3 mason jars.

5. Add a teaspoon of turmeric to each of the jar, mix and add 1-2 lemon slices.

Nutritional Information Per Serving

Calories - 70, Carbohydrates - 1g, Fat - 4g, Proteins - 6g

Almond Butter

Can be eaten alone or in combination with other foods.

Preparation time: 10 minutes

Cooking time: 20 minutes

Servings: 16

Ingredients:

7 1/2 ounces of blanched almonds

1 tablespoon of coconut oil

A pinch of salt

Directions:

1. Preheat oven to 300°F.

2. Roast the almonds for 20 minutes. Stir a few times to ensure they do not burn. Allow to cool

3. Process the almonds and salt in a food processor until it looks like butter.

4. Add the coconut butter and process for a few minutes.

Nutritional Information Per Serving

Calories - 112, Carbohydrates - 1.2g, Fat - 7.4g, Proteins - 2.8, Fiber - 1.3g

Keto Pesto

Serve it on anything!

Preparation time: 10 minutes

Cooking time: 0 minutes

Servings: 16

Ingredients:

2 cups of fresh basil

1/2 cup of olive oil

1/3 cup of pine nuts

1/3 cup of Parmesan cheese

2 garlic cloves

1/2 teaspoon of salt

1/4 teaspoon of black pepper

Directions:

1. Process all the ingredients in a food processor until smooth.

2. Store in a mason jar and refrigerate.

Nutritional Information Per Serving

Calories - 100, Carbohydrates - 0.5, Fat - 9g, Proteins - 4.5g

Caesar Dressing

Bring your salads to life with this dressing.

Preparation time: 5 minutes

Cooking time: 0 minutes

Servings: 16

Ingredients:

3/4 cup of mayonnaise

2 tablespoons of lemon juice, freshly squeezed

3 garlic cloves, finely crushed

1 ½ teaspoons of anchovy paste

1 ½ teaspoons of Dijon mustard

1 teaspoon of Worcestershire sauce

Salt

Pepper

Directions:

1. In a bowl, whisk all the ingredients together thoroughly.

2. Store in a mason jar.

Nutritional Information Per Serving

Calories - 100.39, Carbohydrates - 0.51g, Fat - 10.74g, Proteins - 0.54g

Ranch Dressing

Have this flavor at home at all times.

Preparation time: 2 minutes

Cooking time: 0 minutes

Servings: 20

Ingredients:

1 cup of mayonnaise

¼ cup of heavy whipping cream

½ cup of sour cream

2 tablespoons of dried parsley

½ teaspoon of garlic granules

½ teaspoon of dried dill

½ teaspoon of onion powder

¼ teaspoon of pepper

¼ teaspoon of basil

Directions:

1. Process all the ingredients in an emulsion blender for about a minute until smooth.

2. Store in a mason jar and keep refrigerated.

Nutritional Information Per Serving

Calories - 105.5g, Carbohydrates - 0.57g, Fat - 11.29g, Proteins - 0.65g

Vegan Ranch Dressing

Preparation time: 10 minutes

Cooking time: 0 minutes

Servings: 12

Ingredients:

1/2 cup of vegan mayo

1/2 cup of hemp seeds, hulled

1/2 cup of water

2-3 tablespoons of fresh parsley, chopped

2-3 tablespoons of fresh dill, chopped

1/2 tsp garlic powder

1 tsp onion powder

Salt

Pepper

Directions:

1. Blend the water, onion, hempseeds, garlic and salt in a blender until smooth.

2. Add the mayo, parsley, dill, pepper and blend to mix.

3. Transfer to an airtight jar and keep refrigerated.

Nutritional Information Per Serving

Calories - 109, Carbohydrates - 0g, Fat - 9.9g, Proteins - 2.5g, Fiber - 8g

Coconut Butter

You cannot beat the flavors!

Preparation time: 5 minutes

Cooking time: 0 minutes

Servings: 10

Ingredients:

5 ounces of coconut or coconut chips, shredded

A pinch of salt

Directions:

1. Process the coconut in a food processor until it achieves its desired consistency.

2. Transfer to a jar and keep refrigerated.

Nutritional Information Per Serving

Calories - 102, Carbohydrates - 3.2g, Fat - 9.7g, Proteins - 0.8g, Fiber - 0g

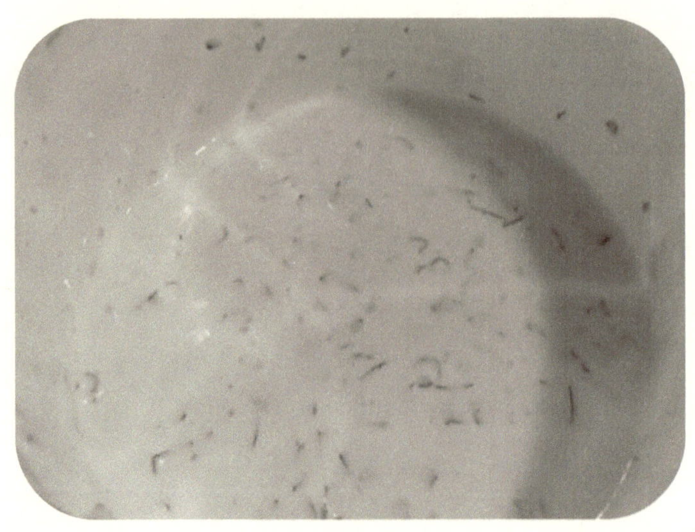

Ranch Dressing

Macadamia Pumpkin Butter

Snack on this whenever you want.

Preparation time: 10 minutes

Cooking time: 0 minutes

Servings: 8

Ingredients:

10 drops of liquid stevia

2 cups of pumpkin seeds

1 cup of macadamia nuts

1/4 teaspoon of sea salt

Directions:

1. In a food processor, process all the ingredients until creamy and smooth.

2. If preferred, adjust taste.

3. Store in a mason jar and keep refrigerated.

Nutritional Information Per Serving

Calories - 300, Carbohydrates - 2g, Fat - 27g, Proteins - 10g

Keto Mayo

Healthy, easy and has no carbs.

Preparation time: 10 minutes

Cooking time: 0 minutes

Servings: 8

Ingredients:

3/4 cup of avocado oil

3 tablespoons of apple cider vinegar

Juice of 1/2 lemon

1 egg yolk

1/2 teaspoon of sea salt

1/4 teaspoon of garlic powder

1/4 teaspoon of paprika

Directions:

1. Process all the ingredients except the oil in a food processor for about a minute.

2. Add about a tablespoon of oil through the processor opening while it is still running. Pause for a bit between each adding so that the oil can emulsify.

3. Transfer the mixture to a mason jar once it has emulsified. Keep refrigerated.

Nutritional Information Per Serving

Calories - 95, Carbohydrates - 0g, Fat - 11g, Proteins - 0g, Fiber - 0g

Conclusion

Many people, having achieved their desired weight goal, usually want to stay off the keto diet. If you are one of these people, I would like to congratulate you on this success, and then to say that if you'd want to go off keto diet, you are free to do so.

Have it in mind however, that if you return to your old eating habits and lifestyle, you will regain your weight. To avoid this, you need to keep your intake in check, so you don't eat excessively and store it as fat. The great thing about sticking to a low carb, high fat diet is that it makes you feel generally great!

www.ingramcontent.com/pod-product-compliance
Lightning Source LLC
Chambersburg PA
CBHW031111250726
48655CB00004B/1663